Michelle Melgarejo da Rosa

Hospital Pharmacy - a view from undergraduate pharmacy students

Michelle Melgarejo da Rosa

Hospital Pharmacy - a view from undergraduate pharmacy students

Nine fields of action for Hospital Pharmacists in the view of UNIFBV-Wyden Pharmacy students

ScienciaScripts

Imprint
Any brand names and product names mentioned in this book are subject to trademark, brand or patent protection and are trademarks or registered trademarks of their respective holders. The use of brand names, product names, common names, trade names, product descriptions etc. even without a particular marking in this work is in no way to be construed to mean that such names may be regarded as unrestricted in respect of trademark and brand protection legislation and could thus be used by anyone.

Cover image: Provided by the author

This book is a translation from the original published under ISBN 978-613-9-79362-4.

Publisher:
Sciencia Scripts
is a trademark of
Dodo Books Indian Ocean Ltd. and OmniScriptum S.R.L publishing group

120 High Road, East Finchley, London, N2 9ED, United Kingdom
Str. Armeneasca 28/1, office 1, Chisinau MD-2012, Republic of Moldova, Europe
Printed at: see last page
ISBN: 978-620-6-41621-0

Chapters and authors:

Chapters presented to the Hospital Pharmacy course at the FBV-Wyden University Centre. Responsible professor and reviewer: Dr Michelle Melgarejo da Rosa

Chapter 1
PHARMACOVIGILANCE: HISTORY AND EVOLUTION IN BRAZIL

Alessandra Karla Souza Lins[1] , Michelle Melgarejo da Rosa[2]

1 - Pharmacy student at UniFBV Wyden University Centre

2 - Professor of Pharmacy at UniFBV Wyden University Centre

The first Adverse Drug Reactions (ADRs) have been reported since ancient times. In 2200 BC, the Babylonian Code of Hammurabi stated that if a doctor caused the death of a patient, their hand would be amputated.

The first record of ADRs was in 1848, which marked the beginning of the institutional framework for pharmacovigilance. A 15-year-old girl underwent surgery and ended up suffering fibrillation as a result of the anaesthetic used (chloroform), leading to the patient's death (VARALLO; MASTROIANNI, 2011).

In 1961, a German paediatrician observed a link between the use of the drug Thalidomide in the first trimester of pregnancy and the birth of babies with congenital malformations (phocomelia). At the same time, there were already at least 300 cases of thalidomide-related phocomelia in Brazil.

Adverse events are damage to the patient's or user's health and can be seen during treatment with pharmaceutical products. They are related to medication errors, adverse drug reactions (ADRs), drug interactions and intoxication (PRATA MENDES et al., 2008).

In 1968, the World Health Organisation (WHO) set up a Pilot Drug Monitoring Programme, in which ten countries took part. The aim was to standardise a national system for reporting adverse reactions.

In 1969, the WHO published standard 425, which conceptualised pharmacovigilance as a set of procedures for detecting, recording and evaluating adverse events to determine their incidence, severity and the causal relationship between the use of the drug and the appearance of the adverse effect. Currently, the World Health Organisation's Drug Safety Programme is coordinated by the Uppsala Monitoring Center, located in Sweden under the supervision of an international committee. Its main objective is to manage the international database of ADR reports received from national centres, as well as to create effective methods for detecting adverse events not revealed in clinical studies. In 1992, pharmacovigilance was formally introduced into the research and academic world (VARALLO; MASTROIANNI, 2011).

In 2002, the World Health Organisation (WHO) expanded the concept of pharmacovigilance, adding it as a science related to the detection, evaluation, understanding and prevention of adverse effects or any problem related to medicines. Its main objective is to guarantee patient safety and the rational use of these medicines (PEZATO; CESARETTI, 2015).

PHARMACOVIGILANCE IN BRAZIL

In the 1970s, the first issues related to adverse reactions arose. Some legislation was published, but it was considered unsuccessful in the development of pharmacovigilance (PRATA MENDES et al., 2008).

In 1995, the first meeting was held to draw up strategies for the implementation of pharmacovigilance systems in Latin America.

In 1998, the National Medicines Policy was approved, its main objective being to guarantee the necessary safety, efficacy and quality of medicines, the promotion of rational use and access to those considered essential (PRATA MENDES et al., 2008).

Almost 25 years later, pharmacovigilance is beginning to be consolidated in Brazil, with the implementation of the National Medicines Policy, the founding of the National Health Surveillance Agency (ANVISA), the creation of the National Centre for Monitoring Medicines, the creation of the Sentinel Network Project, and Brazil's inclusion as a member of the WHO's International Medicines Monitoring Programme in 2001 (PAGOTTO et al., 2013).

The pharmacovigilance programme in Brazil is a combination of the projects mentioned above, which work in partnership on essential issues concerning the safety, effectiveness, quality and rationality of medicines sold throughout Brazil. The effectiveness of this programme will depend on maintaining the project, training health professionals and raising their awareness of the need to voluntarily report events related to the use of medicines (PRATA MENDES et al., 2008).

In 1999, in addition to the creation of Anvisa, it also created the National Pharmacovigilance System, led by the Pharmacovigilance Unit (UFARM), which is part of the new General Management of Post-Marketing Health Product Safety. UFARM's remit is to plan, coordinate and supervise the entire process of formulating and developing guidelines and technical operating standards on the use and surveillance of medicines. One of UFARM's basic strategies is development at state level with a focus on Health Surveillance, which will form state centres (PRATA MENDES et al., 2008).

Legislation on pharmacovigilance in Brazil

Pharmacovigilance interventions in Brazil were already protected by general legislation, such as Federal Law 6360/76, Federal Law 9782/99, National Health Council Resolution 3/89 and Ministry of Health Ordinance 3916/98. In addition, other legislation relating to medicines required pharmacovigilance data when it came to renewing registration.

In 2009, Anvisa published the first specific pharmacovigilance standard for drug registration holders, Collegiate Board Resolution (RDC) No. 04 of 10 February 2009. In the same year, Normative Instruction (IN) No. 14 of 27 October 2009 published the Pharmacovigilance Guides for drug registration holders related to RDC No. 04. Since the validation of RDC 04, the notification of adverse events related to the use of medicines has been compulsory for all medicine registration holders in Portugal. This established the pharmacovigilance inspection, which will be carried out by the regulatory agency in order to verify the existence of a pharmacovigilance system in pharmaceutical companies, as well as other legal requirements. In addition, it is compulsory to send periodic pharmacovigilance reports (RPF) and pharmacovigilance plans to Anvisa on a regular basis. Anvisa may also require risk minimisation plans in the event of specific cases relating to the safety of medicines. Anvisa has increasingly intensified its post-marketing pharmacovigilance actions. It has published rules establishing notification by health professionals associated with oseltamivir (RDC 45/2009), thalidomide (MS Resolution 11/2011) and sibutramine (RDC 50/2014) (ANVISA).

In addition to the legislation already mentioned, there are several other federal laws, ordinances and resolutions that support pharmacovigilance actions in Brazil. These laws are listed in the table below (ANVISA).

Table: Pharmacovigilance legislation in Brazil. Source: Anvisa, modified.

Other legislation that reinforces pharmacovigilance activities in Brazil	
Ordinance No. 802 of 08 October 1998	It stipulates that in the event of complaints, observations and adverse reactions, distributors must immediately separate the batch and notify the registration holder and the health authority.
Ordinance No. 06 of 29 January 1999	Defines that the local health authority must establish mechanisms for the pharmacovigilance of medicines based on the substances listed in Ordinance SVS/MS No. 344/98 (and updates), establishing a specific model for a pharmacovigilance form for retinoid medicines for systemic use and a form for reporting suspected adverse reactions.
Ordinance of the Ministry of Health No. 696 of 7 May 2001	Establishes the National Medicines Monitoring Centre (CNMM), based at Anvisa's Pharmacovigilance Unit.
Decree No. 3.961, of 10 October 2001	Amends Decree No. 79.094/77, which regulates Law No. 6.360/76, including pharmacovigilance in health surveillance actions, as a way of investigating the effects that compromise the safety, efficacy or risk-benefit ratio of a product.
	Determines that the manufacturer of extracts and allergenic products must have a

Collegiate Board Resolution - RDC no. 233, of 17 August 2005	recording and statistical system for pharmacovigilance studies and that, when clinical experience is available , the data is analysed and analysed. pharmacotoxicological studies should be replaced by pharmacovigilance studies or clinical trials.
Collegiate Board Resolution - RDC No. 67, of 8 October 2007	Defines the role of the pharmacist in the compounding pharmacy as participating in pharmacovigilance studies and informing the health authorities of the occurrence of adverse events and/or unforeseen drug interactions.
Ordinance No. 1660 of 22 July 2009	Establishes the Sanitary Surveillance Notification and Investigation System - Vigipos, within the scope of the National Sanitary Surveillance System, as an integral part of the Unified Health System - SUS.
Collegiate Board Resolution - RDC No. 44, of 17 August 2009	Establishes that pharmacists in pharmacies and drugstores must contribute to pharmacovigilance by reporting the occurrence or suspicion of an adverse event or technical complaint to the health authorities.
Collegiate Board Resolution - RDC n°47, of 8 September 2009	Determines that Anvisa may require changes to the texts of package leaflets, whenever it deems it necessary, on the basis of information arising from the pharmacovigilance.
Resolution - RDC No. 60, of 26 April	Establishes that the procedures adopted for the notification of adverse events to

November 2009	medicines must be the same for the free samples.
Collegiate Board Resolution - RDC No. 64, of 18 December 2009	The documentation for the registration of radiopharmaceuticals includes the submission of an updated Pharmacovigilance Report, in accordance with current legislation, with data obtained from clinical studies and from the marketing of the product in other countries, where applicable. For registration renewal, pharmacovigilance data must be submitted. This data may be requested by Anvisa before the deadlines set.
Collegiate Board Resolution - RDC No. 49, of 20 September 2011	Requires the submission of the Periodic Pharmacovigilance Report, the Pharmacovigilance Plan and the Risk Minimisation Plan in specific situations related to drug safety when renewing the registration of biological medicines.
Collegiate Board Resolution - RDC No. 26 of 13 May 2014	It includes the company's Pharmacovigilance System Description Document in the documentation for the registration of herbal medicines. For registration renewal, the requirements of RDC 04/2009 must be followed.
Ordinance No. 650 of 29 May 2014	Approves and promulgates the Internal Regulations of the National Health Surveillance Agency - Anvisa and other measures.

PHARMACOVIGILANCE IN THE HOSPITAL ENVIRONMENT

Medicines are essential in health care, as they provide patients with a better quality of life, whether for prophylactic, curative, palliative or diagnostic purposes. However, their use can pose risks of unwanted effects, which can cause damage ranging from prolonged hospitalisation, the need for diagnostic and therapeutic interventions, or even lead to the patient's death (DUARTE; BATISTA; ALBUQUERQUE, 2014).

In the USA, it is estimated that around 100,000 people die in hospital each year as a result of adverse drug reactions, making it the fourth leading cause of death. This can result in a higher mortality rate than patients with HIV, breast cancer or car accidents (DUARTE; BATISTA; ALBUQUERQUE, 2014).

In Brazil, the epidemiology of Adverse Drug Reactions (ADRs) has been little investigated. Some studies show that health professionals still have great difficulty in making notifications. Pharmacists are still the ones who register the most notifications, ranking first with 50% of notifications, nurses with 37.5%, nursing technicians 17.2 and doctors are the ones who report the least, as a study carried out at the University Hospital/UFJE found that of the five doctors who were on duty and were interviewed, none reported ADRs (LIMA et al., 2014).

Several factors can lead to the appearance of adverse drug reactions, such as age, sex, gender, concomitant use of drugs, among others. Some can have a more direct influence on the onset of ADRs, while others are insidious. This requires greater attention from health professionals (MODESTO et al., 2016).

With the aim of improving and systematising the surveillance of supplies used in the healthcare network, guaranteeing greater quality and safety for patients and healthcare professionals, Anvisa has created the Sentinel Network project in partnership with the largest hospitals in Brazil. One of the main objectives of the Sentinel Network is to increase the number of reports, as well as to educate health professionals by expanding the base of reports to include pharmacists and nurses, active searches in the various sectors of the hospital, the introduction of electronic links to facilitate reporting via the internet, and the aim of improving reports through personalised communications or periodic bulletins (LIMA S. PRISCILA., AZEVEDO C. C. RITA., 2014).

In view of the above, we can see that there has been a great evolution in the history of pharmacovigilance, from its recognition as a science to the creation of legislation that supports it. However, there is still a certain amount of resistance on the part of health professionals to reporting possible ADRs. Projects such as the Sentinel Network need to be maintained in order to better train health professionals and sensitise them to reporting.

REFERENCES

DUARTE, M. L.; BATISTA, L. M.; ALBUQUERQUE, P. M. S. Notifica^oes de Farmacovigilancia em um Hospital Oncologico Sentinela da Paraiba. **Rev. Bras. Pharm. Hosp. Serv. Saude Sao Paulo** , v. 5, n. 1, p. 7-11, 2014.

LIMA S. PRISCILA, AZEVEDO C. C. RITA., DA L. A. DE A. A. Pharmacovigilance: Knowledge and Action of the Professionals Facing the Deviations of Quality of Medicines Pharmacovigilance: Knowledge and Action of the Professionals Facing the Deviations of Quality of Medicines Pharmacovigilance: Knowledge and Action of L. **Original Article Rev. Bras. Pharm. Hosp. Serv**, v. 5 n.1, p. 33-37, 2014.

MODESTO, A. C. F. et al. Adverse Drug Reactions and Pharmacovigilance: Knowledge and Behaviour of Health Professionals at a Sentinel Network Hospital. **Revista Brasileira de Educa^ao Medica**, v. 40, n. 3, p. 401-410, 2016.

PAGOTTO, C. et al. RESULTS OF EDUCATIONAL INTERVENTIONS IN PHARMACOVIGILANCE: 2013.

PEZATO, T. P. J.; CESARETTI, M. L. R. Hospital pharmacovigilance: the importance of training professionals to maximise their actions. **Revista da Faculdade de Ciencias Medicas de Sorocaba**, v. 17, n. 3, p. 135-139, 2015.

PRATA MENDES, M. C. et al. Pharmacovigilance history in Brazil Pharmacovigilance history in Brazil. **Rev. Bras. Farm**, v. 89, n. 3, p. 246-251, 2008.

VARALLO, F. R.; MASTROIANNI, P. C. **Farmacovigilancia**, 2013.

ANVISA. National Health Surveillance Agency (ANVISA).

Chapter 2

PHARMACOVIGILANCE APPLIED TO HOSPITAL PHARMACY

Lucielle Rayane Cosme da Silva[1] ; Michelle Melgarejo da Rosa[2]

1 - Pharmacy student at UniFBV Wyden University Centre

2 - Professor of Pharmacy at UniFBV Wyden University Centre

Pharmacovigilance aims to identify, evaluate, understand and prevent adverse effects or any problems related to the use of medicines (ANVISA, 2018). Adverse drug reactions (ADRs) are one of the biggest problems in hospital settings and are also one of the main causes of increased mortality. This situation can be aggravated by drug interactions, which are facilitated by polypharmacy - a term used when several different drugs are administered concomitantly for the prolonged treatment of a patient - a condition that is increasingly common among the elderly, for example (Mashaba TP, 2018). Pharmacovigilance is responsible for establishing the pharmacological characteristics of medicines before they are marketed, as well as for analysing the possible occurrence of adverse events in medicines already on the market (Hosohata K, 2018). There are various methods that can be used to implement pharmacovigilance, including projects aimed directly at the treatment process and therefore at preventing and/or reducing ADRs. In order to ensure that the benefits of using these medicines outweigh the risks they cause.

The role of the pharmacist should not only be limited to the supervision of medicines and adverse effects, there are other relevant issues that are part of pharmacovigilance and should be taken into account by this professional, such as therapeutic ineffectiveness and medication errors within the hospital context (AlShammari TM, 2018). In order to prevent this important clinical problem, it is necessary to practise actions through a rational distribution system, aiming for improvements such as dispensing by unit dose, enabling the patient to receive the medicine in the correct dose and at the correct time. It is also advisable to create a medicines information centre (CIM) in the hospital environment, with the priority goal of making this sector a disseminator of information on medicines to the multiprofessional health team (Mendes D, 2018). In order to receive and monitor news about incidents, adverse effects and technical complaints related to the use of medicines, the National Health Surveillance Agency (ANVISA) has created a single notification channel (NOTIVISA). It should be made clear that it is not only the pharmacist who can make these notifications, they should be made by any health professional. Pharmacovigilance is an expensive activity, as it requires a good infrastructure and data support from the hospital, as well as skilled professionals who are able to take an active role in the improvement process together with the multi-professional team. This is the only disadvantage that prevents it from being adopted by more and more hospitals, but if you make a brief cost-benefit analysis, its advantages outweigh them. Once it is set up, it becomes indispensable and very rewarding, considering that if there is early detection of adverse effects and determination of the factors that predispose to the appearance of ADRs, the costs of hospitalisation and treatment for adverse events will decrease substantially, as will the rates of poisoning and the use of medicines for indications not previously approved on the register (Bahnassi A, 2018). The success of programmes like the CIM depends exclusively on the adoption and commitment of the team, so that each adverse reaction can be reported, described and then evaluated by everyone, with the aim of ensuring that events like these do not happen again or that, in the event of new occurrences, everyone knows what to do. With this, it is hoped that over time the multi-professional team will be increasingly integrated into this pharmacovigilance method, making it part of the hospital's routine and normal flow.

Depending on the number of cases reported, it will be possible to investigate causality and identify drug safety problems. After all these observations about this method, it is of fundamental importance to understand a little about others that can also be used. The intensive monitoring method is quite common and is one of the most widely used in hospitals. In addition to information on adverse reactions, it is possible to add clinical notes on the patient's condition, intoxications and whether they are allergic to any other medication. It is also capable of producing studies according to population group and linking them to a suspected drug that has greater evidence of ADRs (Ngunyen KD, 2018). This can even identify unexpected reactions that would theoretically not be related to the use of the drug, which is important for polymedicated patients, such as the elderly and those with chronic diseases (Mashaba TP, 2018).

As it has a greater focus on the clinical area, it is the most complete method that can be used in pharmacovigilance. On the other hand, it is more complex and has an excessive cost compared to other existing methods, which ends up making it difficult to use in hospital practice, even though it is very important. The third most widely used method is also the simplest and has a low cost of implementation; it can be said that the pharmacovigilance observational study method, as the name implies, is concerned only with analysing observations, without professionals making any subsequent intervention with the data obtained. It therefore corresponds to a case-control study (Li x 2018). There is also a method that is little used but should also be explained. The prescription correlation system, which is based not only on reported cases of ADRs, but on probable events that may occur induced by the same drug. As previously mentioned, this method is not widely used in clinical practice, but it is quite common to use it for out-of-hospital cross-sectional studies because they only monitor their specific environment (Thompson Um, 2018). However, it is of the utmost importance that in all methods, cause and effect relationships are defined between known adverse reactions and suspected drugs, so that any professional accessing hospital data can clearly and cohesively identify the data present there. In general, methods can be divided into two groups of studies, standardised and non-standardised. Standardised methods are those that were created by applying questionnaires to identify the main causalities and what they had in common with ADRs caused by a particular group of drugs. Non-standardised study methods, on the other hand, allow a different diagnosis to be made for each patient, taking into account their individuality and clinical condition, without pre-established questionnaires or any other comparisons with previous cases (Usui M, 2018).

Pharmacists are the most qualified professionals to design and implement these programmes, as they have a greater command of pharmacokinetics and pharmacodynamics. But this is not the only reason why they are vital to the hospital's development, as they will work in a number of areas, ensuring that patients receive the right treatment in the right conditions, at the right dose for their needs, reducing the abuse of drugs and consequently reducing the hospital's expenditure on effective therapy. Furthermore, they can act after the incidence of ADRs, providing support to the team on the pharmacokinetics and pharmacodynamics of the drugs and to the patient, with pharmaceutical care. One of the most important focuses of hospital pharmacists within their team is minimising errors, which in some cases can be avoided because they are predictable. It was found that the greatest number of cases of adverse reactions are in patients who have been hospitalised for a long time, so there are already some signs and symptoms that may be associated with a series of ADRs that are common in these conduits, which is why it is essential to be alert at all times in order to reduce the number of notifications due to negligence.

While providing pharmaceutical care at the bedside, the pharmacist should gather as much information as possible in order to look for reasons why the pharmacist had such a reaction; apart from age, the most common causes were allergies, kidney and liver dysfunctions (Falconer N, 2018). It is crucial that pharmacists working in pharmacovigilance have extensive knowledge of applied pharmacology and the interpretation of laboratory tests. In addition, pharmacists must be aware of the toxicological potential of each drug that presents adverse reactions with greater frequency. Due to the rational system of dispensing medicines by unit dose, the pharmacist now has greater power over the entry and exit of medicines within the hospital, knowing, for example, whether or not the medicine has been administered to the patient, whether there has been an unexpected suspension of the medication or a reduction in the dose. It is also possible to find out if interchangeability has occurred, an event such as this, despite appearing quite simple and without any major apparent problems, can be a probable cause of ADR (Falconer N, 2018).

It is also worth highlighting two important causes of intercession that predispose to severe reactions: drug-nutrient interaction, where it is common for nutrition, whether enteral or parenteral, to alter the pharmacokinetics of the drug, causing unexpected reactions for the patient's situation, as well as the interaction of the drug with secondary pathologies that are not being treated. These situations have recurred in the prescribing of antihistamines, corticosteroids and antidotes. Understanding everything that has been said so far, it is essential that we also understand that the pharmacovigilance sector needs to have a direct link with the hospital quality control sector, so that it can certify the quality of the services that have been provided to the patient and ensure that the good conditions of the hospital are guaranteed.

REFERENCES

National Health Surveillance Agency. **Pharmacovigilance**. Available at: <http://portal.anvisa.gov.br/farmacovigilancia>. Accessed on: Nov 2018.

AlShammari TM; Almoslem MJ. **Knowledge, attitudes and practices of healthcare professionals in hospitals for reporting adverse drug reactions in Saudi Arabia: A multicentre cross-sectional study.** Saudi Pharm J. Nov 2018.

Bahnassi A; Al-Harbi F. **Syrian pharmacovigilance system: a survey of pharmacists' knowledge, attitudes and practices.** East Mediterr Health J. Jul 2018.

Dastan F; Jamaati H; Emami H; Haghgoo R; Eskandari R; Hashemifard SS; Khoddami F; Mirshafieli Langari Z. **Reducing inappropriate albumin utilisation: the value of the pharmacist-led intervention model.** Ira j Pharm Res. Mar 2018.

Falconer N; Barras M; Martin J; Cottrell N. **Defining and categorising terminology for medication harm: a call for consensus.** Eur J Clin Pharmacol. Oct 2018.

Hosohata K; Matsuoka E; Inada Um; Oyama S; Niinomi l; Mori Y; YamaguchiY; Uchida M; Iwanaga K. **Differential profiles of adverse events associated with mycophenolate mofetil among adult and paediatric renal transplant patients.** J Int Med Res. Nov 2018.

Li x; Thai S; Lu W; Sun; Tang H; Zhai S; Wang T. **Traditional Chinese medicine and drug-induced anaphylaxis: data from the Beijing pharmacovigilance database.** Int J Clin Pharm. Aug

2018.

Mashaba TP; Matlata M; Godman B; Meyer JC. **Implementation and monitoring of decisions by pharmacy and therapeutics committees in public sector hospitals in South Africa.** Expert Rev Clin Pharmacol. Nov 2018.

Mendes D; Alves; Loureiro M; Fonte A; Batel-Marques F. **Drug-induced hypersensitivity: A 5-year retrospective study in an electronic database of hospital records.** J Clin Pharm Ther. Aug 2018.

Ngunyen KD; Tran TN; Nguyen MT; Ngunyen HA; Nguyen HA Jr; DH Vu; Nguyen VD; Bagheri H. **Drug-induced Stevens-Johnson syndrome and toxic epidermal necrolysis in a spontaneous adverse drug reaction database from Vietnam: A subgroup approach to disproportionality analysis.** J Clin Pharm Ther. Aug 2018.

Terblancle A; Meyer JC; Godman B; Verdes RS. **Impact of a pharmacist-led pharmacovigilance system in a secondary hospital in Gauteng Province, South Africa.** Hosp Pract (1995). Oct 2018.

Thompson Um; Randall C; Howard J; Barker C; Bowden D; Mooney P; Munyika Um; Smith S; Pirmohamed M. **Non-prescribed experiences in doctor training and competency to report adverse drug events in the UK.** J Clin Pharm Ther. Sep 2018.

Usui M; Aramaki E; Iwao T; Wakamiya S; Sakamoto T; Mochizuki M. **Extraction and Standardisation of Patient Complaints from Electronic Medication Histories for Pharmacovigilance: Natural Language Processing Analysis in Japanese.** JMIR Med Inform. Sep 2018.

Xie X; Jin X; Zhang L; Sol H; Shen A; Huang X; Sol Y. **Trend analysis for medication utilisation in county public hospitals: a sample study from the pilot area in healthcare reform in China.** BMC Health Serv Res. Oct 2018.

Zhao Y; Wang T; Li G; Sun S. **Pharmacovigilance in China: development and challenges.** Int J Clin Pharm. Aug 2018.

Chapter 3
THE PHARMACIST IN HOSPITAL HEALTH SURVEILLANCE

Danyely Santos[1] , Cleciane Salvador[1] , Michelle Melgarejo da Rosa[2]

1 - Pharmacy student at UniFBV Wyden University Centre

2 - Professor of Pharmacy at UniFBV Wyden University Centre

Health surveillance is a public sector body that promotes actions aimed at preventing, eliminating or reducing health risks, on a state, municipal and national scale. The sanitary pharmacist is a professional who, according to their training, is able to work in the sanitary sector, acting in conjunction with the multi-professional team to promote measures to prevent health risks and inspect establishments (SOUSA, B. et al., 2017).

Because of their training and knowledge of the related legislation, pharmacists are the only professionals who have the technical capacity to monitor any health risks related to the manufacture, storage, handling, transport and distribution of drugs, supplies and health products. The sanitary pharmacist can work in various sectors, such as drugstores, handling pharmacies, public pharmacies, hospital pharmacies, drug distributors, drug importers/exporters and drug industries, all of which are registered with the Federal Pharmacy Council (CFF). Other sectors can be inspected by the pharmacist, such as: industries (sanitisers/food), disinsecticides, clinical analysis laboratories, among others. Professional pharmacists will only be able to carry out these duties if they meet the conditions laid down in Resolution 539 of 22 October 2010 of the Federal Pharmacy Council (Brazil). This chapter will focus on the role of the pharmacist in Health Surveillance and actions within hospitals, demonstrating their role and importance.

Concept of health surveillance

Surveillance is part of a large system of supervision and organisation, and its practices are present in a wide range of environments, whether hospital, food, environmental, agronomic, civil construction, naval, veterinary or many others. All with the aim of preventing risks and promoting the health of living beings, reducing and/or eliminating problems that may interfere with the common good of society; with services that analyse everything from the construction of a structure to the hygiene conditions of a neighbourhood snack bar.

For hospital, clinical or everyday health practices (airports, hotels, cafeterias, etc.), there is the Sanitary Surveillance (VISA), currently a state and municipal body, which operates within the

National Sanitary Surveillance System (SNVS), which is responsible for monitoring and linking all the VISA bodies in the country, so that they work in a unified way while offering quality and meeting the specific needs of each different region. The SNVS is joined by ANVISA, the National Health Surveillance Agency (coordinator of the SNVS), which is responsible for establishing rules, regulations and laws that must be complied with by the Health Surveillance directorates, as well as contributing financially to their practices and duties.

All of these (VISA, SNVS and ANVISA) are directly linked to the Unified Health System (SUS) and the Ministry of Health, with the aim of being integrated and decentralised throughout Brazil. It is worth emphasising that the services provided by VISA are not only available to the public sector, but also to the private sector, both in equal measure. In other words, the right to good health surveillance is available to everyone, regardless of social class or work environment.

Unfortunately, the idea has been created that the role of health surveillance is limited to closing and interdicting establishments or inspecting expired and spoilt products. However, in addition to these actions, it can act in any way that threatens or harms the health of the target public. According to ANVISA, "its activities cover all market segments directly or indirectly related to health" (BRASIL, 1999).

On ships, for example, they work with the health of passengers and staff. As well as food inspections, there are inspections of water for recreational use, ventilation and air conditioning systems, vector control, solid waste analysis and the provision of PPE and CPE for staff (the only difference with passengers). In hospitals, it can be present in the assessment of the hygiene conduct of inpatients with or without mastery of basic autonomous activities. In markets, it inspects products on the shelf and in the fridge, taking into account expiry dates, damage to packaging, storage and consumption behaviour.

In general, inspections are carried out with the help of standardised forms for each type of service. At the end of the visits, the establishments are given grades which determine their level of quality. A grade, approved establishments meeting 90 per cent or more of the requirements; B grade, establishments assessed as meeting between 80 and 90 per cent of the requirements; C grade, establishments in acceptable conditions, with only 70 per cent compliance with the rules; and D grade, with values below 70 per cent, acting in unsatisfactory conditions, subject to two courses of action: immediate and determined closure or temporary closure for improvement.

This means that the Health Surveillance Service is involved in the smooth running of mutual health, as well as in the day-to-day running of society, as it works assiduously on the infinite number of products and conveniences used or consumed by the population, all to guarantee the quality and safety of the individual.

In other words, according to article 6, paragraph 1, of Law No. 8.080, of 19 September 1990, the following applies:

Health surveillance is understood to be a set of actions capable of eliminating, reducing or preventing risks to health and intervening in health problems arising from the environment, the production and circulation of goods and the provision of services of interest to health:

I. The control of consumer goods that are directly or indirectly related to health, including all stages and processes, from production to consumption (BRASIL, 1990);

II. Control of the provision of services that are directly or indirectly related to health (BRASIL, 1990).

History of Health Surveillance

Activities related to sanitary surveillance arose from the need to control the spread of transmissible diseases in urban centres that lacked sanitary conduits. The literature shows that since ancient times there have been reports of deaths from diseases that we now know were caused by sanitary problems. In the Middle Ages the processes of contamination that spread the diseases that ravaged the cities at the time were not yet known, such as cholera, variola, typhoid fever and others; But even without the specific knowledge of disease transmission, it was known at the time that water and food could be a means of contamination and spread of disease, so it was believed that dangerous outbreaks of disease could arise, slightly in places where food was sold, and so the authorities of the time began to police the market square to prevent the sale of adulterated or spoilt food.

In Europe, ships and their cargoes were inspected when they arrived in harbours in order to prevent the entry of diseases that plagued the regions at the time. Literature shows that activities related to health surveillance date back to around the 17th and 18th centuries in Europe and the 18th and 19th centuries in Brazil, in response to major health problems suffered at the time (COSTA. A. et al., ANVISA 2002).

With the great advances in discoveries in the areas of bacteriology and therapeutics during World War I and II, there were major changes in the restructuring of health surveillance. Over time and with Brazil's economic growth, the activities pertaining to health surveillance in the country began to be structured and around the 80s, It began to rely on popular participation and to administer the activities devised for the state with a view to consumer rights and the health of the population (SECRETARIA DE SAUDE DO PARANA [s. d.]).d.]).

Measures such as improved water transport and supply, a suitable place to dispose of rubbish and other educational measures to enlighten the population were the first to be taken.

With the implementation of ANVISA (National Sanitary Surveillance Agency), created by Law No. 9.782 of 26 January 1999, this body creates the rules that must be implemented by state and municipal surveillance agencies. It is present throughout the national territory and coordinates ports, airports, borders and customs enclosures. Its institutional purpose is to promote the protection of the population's health through sanitary control. With ANVISA's support, state and municipal surveillance agencies have been organising themselves to take care of all the areas to which they have been assigned.

ANVISA, SNVS and VISA

Even though these organisations work together and integrate, they carry out their activities at different levels. For a better understanding, health surveillance is part of a large group of surveillance activities, such as epidemiological surveillance, agronomic surveillance, haemovigilance, technovigilance, environmental surveillance, etc. All of these are designed to supervise, monitor and improve the health, safety and comfort of the population. Sanitary surveillance, known as VISA, has been present in our history since the Middle Ages, working in public markets with small inspections of merchandise and since then it has improved to the current inspection activities. VISA currently performs its function at state and municipal level, and is monitored by SNVS, the National Health Surveillance System, which operates on a federative basis with the function of linking state and federal states, broadening VISA's operating strategy. The SNVS is coordinated by ANVISA, Brazil's National Health Surveillance Agency, a body founded in 1999 by Provisional Measure 1.791, converted into Law 9.782, published on 26 January of the same year, which, despite being created later, has gained greater strength and leadership, and is now responsible for creating and regulating the rules and legislation followed by the SNVS and VISA, as well as being financially responsible for the services provided by both. In addition, all these organisations are linked to the SUS, the Unified Health System.

The importance of the pharmacist in the multi-professional health surveillance team

In order for the prevention and inspection system to function properly, it is important that all health surveillance professionals work together to optimise the body's functionality, carrying out the actions that are their responsibility according to their area. Pharmacists are the only professionals who, according to their training, are able to deal with the inspection and prevention of health risks and damage to health, when it comes to the manufacture, storage, handling, transport and distribution of drugs, supplies and health products. The areas that the pharmacist is responsible for supervising are determined as having a high degree of health risk according to Anvisa's RDC No 153 of 27 April 2017, so the professional's work is indispensable for supervision and licensing. The specific duties of the pharmacist in health surveillance are listed in Federal Laws 13.021/14 and 3.820/1960 and Federal Decree 85.878/1981, which specify the areas in which the pharmacist works exclusively.

Being able to supervise a wide range of products and services, the pharmacist stands out in health surveillance because he is a strategic professional with extensive knowledge, making him versatile for public health.

It is notable that pharmacists are gaining more and more space and recognition for their work, and the inclusion of this professional within the health surveillance team is an advance for public health. They can contribute with their specific knowledge and work together with the multi-professional team to achieve good results and thus promote and protect the health of the population.

Professional pharmacist practice in health surveillance in accordance with resolutions

For the work of the sanitary pharmacist, the areas of activity and conduct for exercising the actions within their remit are listed in the relevant legislation, laws, decrees and resolutions. BRAZIL. Law No. 3.820, 11 November 1960

- According to this law, in order to practise pharmacy in the country, the professional must be registered with the Regional Pharmacy Council;

BRAZIL. Decree No. 85.878 of 7th April 1981

- According to this decree, the sanitary and technical professional supervision of companies, establishments, sectors, formulations, products, processes and pharmaceutical or pharmaceutical methods is the exclusive responsibility of the sanitary pharmacist (Art. 1, item III). Federal Pharmacy Council (BRAZIL). Resolution No. 539 of 22 October 2010;

- According to this resolution, health pharmacists must be registered with the Regional Pharmacy Council of their respective jurisdiction (Art. 1);

- Pharmacists are exclusively responsible for the professional, sanitary and technical supervision of companies, establishments, sectors, formulations, products, processes and methods that are pharmaceutical or of a pharmaceutical nature, and must maintain direct supervision, with no delegation permitted. (Art. 2);

- The professional, technical and sanitary supervision of pharmacists is the pharmacist's prerogative: (Art. 3);

* Dispensing, fractionation and handling of magisterial medicines, magisterial and pharmacopoeial formulas;

* Manipulation and manufacture of Galenic medicines and pharmaceutical specialities;

* Pharmaceutical industrial establishments where products are manufactured that have therapeutic, anaesthetic or auxiliary diagnostic indications and/or actions, or are capable of creating physical or psychological dependence;

* Organisations, laboratories, sectors or pharmaceutical establishments where quality control and/or

inspection, preliminary analysis, control analysis and tax analysis are carried out on products intended for therapeutic, anaesthetic or auxiliary diagnostic purposes or capable of determining physical or psychic dependence;

* Organisations, laboratories, sectors or pharmaceutical establishments where extraction, purification, quality control, quality inspection, preliminary analysis, control analysis and tax analysis of pharmaceutical ingredients of plant, animal and mineral origin are carried out;

* Warehouses of pharmaceutical products of any kind; of companies, establishments, sectors, formulations, products, processes and methods that are pharmaceutical or of a pharmaceutical nature;

* Drawing up technical reports and carrying out technical-legal expertise related to pharmaceutical or pharmaceutical-related activities, products, formulations, processes and methods;

* Establishments that distribute and/or transport medicines and other pharmaceutical products, including land, air, rail or river transport companies (boats, aeroplanes, ports and airports) that transport pharmaceutical products, substances and medicines subject to special control (SOUSA, B. et al., 2017 p.11-12).

Chart 1: Areas of activity of the health pharmacist.

Raw materials and inputs pharmacists	Health products/correlates	Sa nguee haemoderivatives	Cosmetics and medicines	Control of pests
Industrialised or manipulated medicines	Indu stry trade food	Parenteral and enteral nutrition	Chemical analysis laboratories	Treatment and cont rol of wate r quality
Immunobiologicals	Antineoplastics	Agrotoxics	Transport and storage of products of int eresta	Long-stay institutions for the elderly (ILPI)
Medical gases	Radiopharmaceuti cals	Beauty salon	Mortuaries and funeral parlours	Medical, dental and aes thetic clinics hospitals

Sanitisers	Herbal medicines	Hotels	Opticians	Restaurants

Hospital health surveillance

Health inspections in hospitals are carried out according to scripts drawn up by state and/or municipal departments, covering: the hospital structure, materials and waste, sectors of the establishment (ICU, obstetrics, paediatrics, psychiatry, haemodialysis, emergency/urgency, outpatient clinics, reception, etc.), location (longevity and access), HR and management, warehouses, patient transport, hygiene and sterilisation in general, machinery, drug control (pharmacovigilance), biosafety, among others. The operation is carried out by a professional with specialised and proven skills, who can be a health worker, doctors, pharmacists and other health-related professionals (XAVIER, 2007). The importance of this measure is to standardise inspections for certain areas and to assess the quality given by grades: grade A (Sanitary Excellence); grade B (Good sanitary conduct); grade C (Satisfactory, but subject to improvement); and grade D (Unsatisfactory, risk of closure or temporary intervention).

Health surveillance and the hospital

- It takes into account infrastructure, material resources, the layout of the environment, accessibility, air conditioning, driving, machinery and equipment, water quality and toilets for sanitisation, individual and collective protection materials, human and financial resources and the information system.

Health surveillance and the patient/employees

- It takes care of the reception and first consultation in excellence, bed management, cleaning of hospital linen and personal belongings, cleaning of rooms, dormitories and changing rooms, quality food, availability and offer of health services.

Health surveillance and hospital pharmacy

- Drug and pharmacotherapeutic control, outgoing and incoming drugs, industrialised or manipulated, expiry dates, dispensing and filling prescriptions, fraud investigation, stocking supplies (from drugs to dressing materials), filing pharmacotherapies, failures or problems related to drugs.

The importance of hospital pharmacovigilance

According to the World Health Organisation (WHO), pharmacovigilance is defined as "the science and activities relating to the detection, evaluation, understanding and prevention of adverse effects or any other drug-related problem", with the following main objectives: to ensure caution, but also the protection of patients with regard to the use of medicines and any medical intercessions; to improve public health and improve safety in relation to the use of medicines; to detect adversities related to the use of medicines and to report any misunderstandings appropriately; helping to analyse the harm, risks, benefits and effectiveness of medicines, preventing harm and maximising benefits; promoting the safe, logical and more efficient use of medicines; and encouraging understanding, education and clinical training in pharmacovigilance and its objective dissemination to the public (CRISTINA et al., 2008; DRESCH, 2006; PAN-AMERICAN HEALTH ORGANISATION, 2011).

References:
BRAZIL. **ANVISA**. Available at: <http://portal.anvisa.gov.br/institucional>. Accessed on: 20 Nov. 2018.

BRAZIL. **Federal** **Constitution.** Available at : <http://www.planalto.gov.br/ccivil_03/leis/L9782.htm>. Accessed on: 20 Nov. 2018.

CRISTINA, M. et al. History of Pharmacovigilance in Brazil. **Revista Brasileira de Farmacia**, v. 89, n. 3, p. 246-251, 2008.

DRESCH, C. Pharmacovigilance and primary health care: a possible and necessary dialogue. **Revista de Aten^ao Primaria a Saude**, v. 9, p. 73-82, 2006.

PAN-AMERICAN HEALTH ORGANISATION. **Good pharmacovigilance practices for the Americas**. 2011.

XAVIER, R. **VIGILANCIA SANITARIA EM SERVICOS DE SAUDE: controle sanitario da farmacia hospitalar**. [s.l.] Federal University of Bahia, 2007.

SOUSA, B. et al. **The pharmacist in health surveillance**, CFF. Brazil, October 2017.

SILVA, W. **In defence of the pharmacist and the National Health Surveillance System.** n° 80. Pharmacia Brasileira- February/March 2011

SECRETARIAT OF HEALTH OF PARANA. **History of Health Surveillance** [n.d.].

COSTA. A. et al. **Cartilha de vigilancia sanitaria**. ANVISA, Brasilia, Aug. 2002.

Chapter 4
PHARMACEUTICAL ASSISTANCE IN TREATMENT ADHERENCE: PHARMACEUTICAL CARE AND HOME CARE

Laura Cabral Peixoto[1] , Vanessa de Albuquerque Brito[1] and Michelle Melgarejo da Rosa[2]

1 - Pharmacy student at UniFBV Wyden University Centre

2 - Professor of Pharmacy at UniFBV Wyden University Centre

Adherence to drug treatment is the key to successful treatment and total patient convalescence. It is from this that the role of the pharmacist in clinical care arises and, more recently, this care has been extended to home care. In this chapter we will discuss the concepts and methodologies used in pharmaceutical care and the factors related to them.

There is more than one concept that can be used to explain adherence, but more generally, it is understood as the use of prescribed medicines or other procedures in at least 80% of their total amount, observing schedules, doses and treatment time. It represents the final stage of what is suggested as the rational use of medicines (Leite, 2003). Some factors are responsible for patient non-adherence, such as: the high cost, lack of access, medicines that require a great deal of effort on the part of the patient, such as adapting their diet, timetable and daily rhythm to comply with the treatment, the type of illness, which will depend a great deal on the way the patient sees their condition and understands their illness.

PHARMACEUTICAL CARE

Pharmaceutical care in the hospital environment - a focus on patient safety

Drug-related problems (DRPs) are common and can result in reduced quality of life and even increased morbidity and mortality. In this context, pharmacy professionals can effectively identify and prevent clinically significant DRPs, as well as helping to increase patient adherence to treatment and achieve other positive clinical results. According to Resolution 300 of January 1997, the main function of the hospital pharmacist is to guarantee the quality of care provided to patients through the safe and rational use of medicines and related products, and their appropriate use for individual and collective health, in terms of care, prevention, teaching and research.

The most frequent drug-related adverse events were recorded in the Harvard Medical Practice Study II, a considerable proportion of which were preventable. In recent years, the considerable increase in the number of studies on patient safety has led to greater knowledge on the subject, confirming its importance as a global problem. With regard to pharmacotherapy, many patients know why they take their medication. However, there is a notorious lack of knowledge about other important aspects, such as the duration of treatment, adverse effects, possible interference from food and other medicines, lifestyle changes and whether or not they should continue treatment with the medicines they were using before hospitalisation.

A study carried out by Lupatini (2013) in a university hospital in Juiz de Fora showed that after the medical consultation, 28% of the interviewees were classified as having good knowledge of the medicines they were using, 17% as regular and 64% as insufficient, while after pharmaceutical dispensation, 5% were good, 87% regular and 7% insufficient. The authors concluded that the results found after dispensation were better than those found during medical consultations, emphasising the important role of pharmacists in guiding patients on the rational use of medicines.

The use of medication by critically ill patients is an example of the complexity of intensive care unit (ICU) care, since patients are generally polymedicated, making pharmacotherapy an important risk factor for the occurrence of adverse events that can contribute negatively to the patient's clinical evolution.

Pharmacists have been incorporated into the multi-professional ICU team with the aim of providing the best patient care, contributing above all to drug monitoring and efficacy evaluation, thus helping to improve patient safety. In this way, the clinical pharmacist's role in day-to-day ICU patient care occurs mainly through active participation in daily clinical visits, providing information support to the medical and nursing team; analysing and monitoring the effectiveness of pharmacotherapy; carrying out drug reconciliation; and preventing, identifying and reporting adverse events.

Due to the scarcity of similar studies in Brazil, the topic also raises the need for a paradigm shift in the contributions of clinical and hospital pharmacists to daily care practice in intensive care units, acting in a collaborative manner in favour of patient safety and quality of care.

Currently, medication errors are a worldwide public health problem, the most serious being prescription errors. Pharmaceutical care prevents prescribing and administration errors, drastically reducing the number of deaths caused by them and increasing adherence and therapeutic efficacy.

Polypharmacy includes at least one drug that is unnecessary to the patient's drug therapy, increasing the risk of drug-related toxicity when there are comorbidities. In addition, the use of potentially inappropriate medication (PIM) for older people, as defined by the Beers criteria, can cause confusion, cognitive impairment, worsening of clinical symptoms and increased mortality.

Adherence to therapy is directly dependent on a number of factors such as polypharmacy, a complex therapeutic regime, cognitive-functional impairment and reduced manual dexterity. The combination of these factors makes non-adherence to drug treatment one of the most common and serious clinical concerns in this population.

According to VIANA et. al. (2017), only around 50% of patients adhere to drug treatment, and these percentages vary from 47% to 100% in the elderly. Reports of non-adherence lead to around 125,000 deaths. The pharmacist must ensure that the patient follows the therapy fully, thus seeking a positive evolution of the clinical condition.

A significant proportion of adverse drug events (ADRs) are estimated to be preventable and therefore the question arises as to whether healthcare professionals are doing enough to prevent ADRs at the time of prescribing or to identify their onset before the reaction becomes potentially serious. The hospital pharmacist plays a crucial role in reducing these events by reviewing prescriptions before dispensing a drug to the patient.

In addition to improving the patient's quality of life, some studies have shown that pharmaceutical care reduces hospital costs related to care for morbidities caused by medication errors, unnecessary polypharmacy in some therapies, avoidable adverse reactions, among others. In a study carried out by Chinthammi (2012) on pharmaceutical care at hospital discharge, 48% of short stays were reduced after pharmaceutical intervention, making it cost-effective. In addition, discharge counselling was more cost-effective in the high-risk elderly population compared to the general population.

Discharge from hospital is a critical transition for patients because after this point their health is less structured and they are often responsible for their own medication management and monitoring. It is therefore important that patients understand what medication they have been prescribed before leaving hospital. In addition, hospital discharge provides pharmacists with an opportunity to detect medication errors during care.

PHARMACEUTICAL HOME CARE

Home pharmaceutical care, also known as home care, is a type of healthcare service that extends beyond hospital care, aiming to improve the quality of life of its patients, since the main target groups are elderly patients, those with degenerative or chronic syndromes and pathologies, and terminally ill patients, and the home would be a place that would bring greater comfort and independence. It is an excellent alternative for both simple cases (bathing, dressing) and more complex procedures, classified as home care. It comprises a set of outpatient activities with defined, programmed objectives that are carried out continuously (Souza, 2004).

The pharmacist is responsible for the control, distribution and dispensation of medicines, pharmacotherapeutic monitoring of the prescription of medicines, checking for possible problems related to them, adverse reactions, drug interactions and the evolution of the patient's clinical condition according to the chosen drug therapy (Olmedilha, 2013). With home care, this responsibility will have the differential of carrying out an adherence plan that is fully adapted to the social and family factors in which the user is inserted, in other words, a procedure centred on the patient and not just on the medication.

A home visit can be understood as the assistance provided by a health professional or team at the user's home, with the aim of assessing their needs, those of their family and the environment in which they live, in order to establish a care plan aimed at recovery or rehabilitation (Olmedilha, 2013).

The pharmacist works together with a multidisciplinary team made up of doctors, nurses, nutritionists, physiotherapists, speech therapists, pharmacists and other specialists, and is of fundamental importance for efficient pharmacotherapeutic treatment, as it encompasses the services of Pharmaceutical Care, Pharmaceutical Assistance, Pharmacovigilance, Clinical Pharmacy and Pharmaceutical Auditing (Planas et al., 2005).

In home pharmaceutical care, all the actions taken with the patient to achieve the therapeutic goal are recorded, including health education, referrals to other health professionals, pharmacotherapy interventions and non-pharmacological measures such as encouraging physical activity and dietary re-education (Barros, 2005). During every home visit, the pharmacist should draw up a care plan with the positive and negative results of the pharmacological treatment, enabling not only the patient, but also their family members or people living in the same household to take part in therapeutic decisions, learn more about their illness, obtain more information and, consequently, comply better with their treatment and obtain better results (Zelmer, 2001; Paulos, 2002).

Home care services comprise four different types of home health care: home care, in-home care, in-home care and home visits. This division is based on Resolution RDC No. 11 of 26 January 2006 and on a document published by the Ministry of Health in 2004 (Brasil, 2006).

Their duties are regulated by Resolution 386/02 of the Federal Pharmacy Council, in which they provide guidance on the use, indication, interactions (drug and food), side effects, medicines via tubes (enteral and nasoenteral), storage, administration and disposal of medicines for the multidisciplinary team, patients and their families. It also manages the storage of medicines and medical materials, ensuring that they reach the patient's home with quality and safety (CRF, 2013).

The pharmacist must establish an ethical relationship between the organisation that hires him/her and the patients who request the Home Care service, including some prerequisites such as: training the patient, family and carer to administer the medication correctly; assessing whether the medical prescriptions are suitable for Home Care, as well as the indication, dose, route and method of administration of the medication; in cases where the first dose of medication is administered at home, the pharmacist should assess together with the doctor, nurse and carer whether the procedure is safe; they should also monitor, through appropriate laboratory tests, whether the drug therapy is responding positively (ASHP, 2000).

Complete documentation of the patient, such as personal data, history of previous pathologies, diagnoses and test results, site of intravenous application, start of drug therapy, profile of prescribed and non-prescribed medications, functional limitations, as well as the entire evolution of the patient's clinical condition, is very important for the pharmacist when it comes to prescribed drug therapy. It is also up to the pharmacist to choose the right products, devices and supplies for the patient's therapy, taking into account the stability and compatibility of the prescribed drugs in the infusion device. A care plan should be drawn up at the start of therapy and reviewed regularly (ASHP, 2000).

The modality of home care services is still not very well known in Brazil, but within all that has been said here we can emphasise that the advantages of home care services include a reduction in the occupation of hospital beds, greater patient comfort, care adapted to the patient's needs and interdisciplinary care. Home care enables greater interaction between the patient and the professionals involved, increasing family acceptance and speeding up the recovery process.

REFERENCES

SOUZA, CR; LOPES, CF; BARBOSA, MA. The contribution of nurses in the context of health promotion through home visits. Revista da UFG, Goiania, v. 6, p. 4-9, dec. 2004.

REGIONAL PHARMACY COUNCIL. Hospital Pharmacy Primer. Hospital Pharmacy Advisory Committee. 2013.

PLANAS, LG., KIMBERLIN, CL., SEGAL, R., BRUSHWOOD, DB., HEPLER, CD., & SCHLENKER, BR. A pharmacist model of perceived responsibility for drug therapy outcomes. Soc Sci Med. 2005.

BARROS JAC. Aten^ao Farmaceutica - step-by-step implementation. Belo Horizonte: Faculty of Pharmacy, 2005.

ZELMER WA. Role of pharmacy organisations in transforming the profession: the case of pharmaceutical care. Pharm Hist. 2001; 43(2- 3):75-85.
ASHP - Guidelines on the pharmacist's role in home care. Am J Health-Sys Pharm. 2000; 57:1250-5.

HOME CARE SERVICE. RDC 11/2006. Rules on the Technical Regulations for the Operation of Home Care Services.

PAULOS C. Applied pharmaceutical care: how to manage routines and information. Sao Paulo: RACINE, 2002. 94 p. Course material for the 12ª Semana RacineAtualiza^ao Tecnica em

Farmacia.LEITE, SN; VASCONCELLOS, MPC.

Adherence to drug therapy: elements for the discussion of concepts and assumptions adopted in the literature. Ciencia & Saude Coletiva, v. 8, p. 775-782, 2003.

DALTON, K; BYRNE, S. Role of the pharmacist in reducing healthcare costs: current insights. Integrated pharmacy research & practice, v. 6, p. 37, 2017.

LUPATINI, EO; MUNCK, AKR; VIEIRA, RCPA. Perceptions of patients in a teaching hospital regarding pharmacotherapy and pharmaceutical guidance on discharge - Rev. Bras. Pharm. Hosp. Serv. Saude Sao Paulo v.5 n.3 28-33, 2014.

CHINTHAMMI, T C; ARMSTRONG, EP; WARHOLAK, TL. A cost-effectiveness evaluation of hospital discharge counselling by pharmacists. Journal of pharmacy practice, v. 25, n. 2, p. 201-208, 2012.

FIDELES, GMA., ALCANTARA-NETO, JMD., PEIXOTO JUNIOR, AA., SOUZA-NETO, PJD., TONETE, TL., SILVA, JEGD., & NERI, EDR. Pharmacist recommendations in an intensive care unit: three-year clinical activities. Revista Brasileira de terapia intensiva, v. 27, n. 2, p. 149-154, 2015.

FEDERAL PHARMACY COUNCIL. Regulates professional practice in pharmacies and hospital units, clinics and health centres of a public or private nature. Resolution no. 300 of 30 January 1997.

COSTA, JM., MARTINS, JM., PEDROSO, LA., BRAZ, CL., & REIS, AM. Optimisation of pharmaceutical care at hospital discharge: implementation of a pharmacotherapeutic guidance and referral service. Rev. Bras. Pharm. Hosp. Serv. Saude, v. 5, n. 1, p. 38-41, 2014.

WOODS, DJ. The role of hospital pharmacists in the prevention of adverse drug reactions. Rev. Bras. Pharm. Hosp. Serv. Saude Sao Paulo v, v. 8, n. 2, p. 4-7, 2017.

LIMA ED, SILVA RG, RICIERI MC AND BLATT CR. Clinical pharmacy in a hospital environment: focus on recording activities. Rev. Bras. Pharm. Hosp. Serv. Saude, 8(4): 1824, 2018.

VIANA, SSC; ARANTES, T; RIBEIRO, SCC. Interventions of the clinical pharmacist in an Intermediate Care Unit for elderly patients. Einstein (Sao Paulo), v. 15, n. 3, p. 283-288,

2 017.

ROSA, MB., PERINI, E., ANACLETO, TA., NEIVA, HM., & BOGUTCHI, T. Errors in hospital prescriptions of high-alert medications. Revista de saude publica, v. 43, n. 3, p. 490498, 2009.

MARQUES LFG, FURTADO IC, DI MONACO LCR. Hospital discharge: a pharmaceutical approach. Course Conclusion Paper (Specialisation) - Racine Institute - Sao Paulo: 2010. Available at: <http://bvsms.saude.gov.br> Accessed on: 15 November 2010
2 018.

Chapter 5
A LOOK AT THE ROLE OF THE PHARMACIST IN
SUS BASIC CARE.

Lidiane Valentim Maciel[1] , Michelle Melgarejo da Rosa[2]

1 - Pharmacy student at UniFBV Wyden University Centre

2 - Professor of Pharmacy at UniFBV Wyden University Centre

The Unified Health System (SUS), implemented in the 1980s and 1990s, has been changing the Brazilian health system. In recent years there has been intensified debate on the development of Health Care Networks, as a strategy for organising the health system that is potentially capable of increasing the performance of the SUS in terms of access, quality and economic efficiency. Ordinance No. 4.279, of 30 December 2010, establishes the guidelines for the organisation of Health Care Networks within the SUS, highlighting that the Health Care Network is organised on the basis of a "clinical management process associated with the use of microeconomic efficiency criteria in the application of resources, through cooperative intergovernmental planning, management and financing, aimed at developing integrated health policy solutions". The organisation of Primary Care (PC) is a top priority for the Ministry of Health. It aims to work on the main challenges for the expansion and consolidation of primary care in the country (Ministerio da Saude Aten^ao Basica). Pharmaceutical care in primary care involves actions that involve the two dimensions of matrix support: clinical-care and technical-pedagogical. The first refers to pharmaceutical care and direct clinical actions for users, either individually or in a shared manner. The second refers to actions that more directly meet the needs of the teams involved in care, through continuing education and other shared actions (Ministerio da Saude Aten^ao Basica). Thus, through clinical practice, pharmacists can guarantee care for users of the system, as well as assisting other health professionals in the rational use of medicines, whether in terms of health promotion, prevention or rehabilitation (Santos et al., 2017). All professional activities carried out by pharmacists in Brazil are regulated by the Federal Pharmacy Council (CFF), based on Law No. 3,820, signed on 11 November 1960.

CFF Resolution No. 578 of 2013 regulates the technical and managerial attributions of pharmacists in the management of pharmaceutical care within the scope of the Unified Health System. This Resolution sets out the guidelines for the relevant role of the pharmacist in health policy, assigning:

• Participate in policy formulation and action planning, in line with the health policy of their sphere of activity and with social control;

- Participating in drawing up the health plan and other management instruments in its sphere of activity;

The pharmacist in SUS pharmaceutical assistance has the following guidelines for action:
- Use control, monitoring and evaluation tools to monitor the health plan and support decision-making in their sphere of activity;
- Participating in the drug selection process;
- Drawing up the programme for the purchase of medicines in its sphere of management;
- Advising on the drafting of calls for tender for the purchase of medicines and other health products and the other stages of the process;
- Participate in the processes of valorisation, training and qualification of health professionals who work in pharmaceutical care;
- Permanently evaluating the existing conditions for the storage, distribution and dispensation of medicines, making the necessary referrals to comply with current health legislation;
- Develop actions to promote the rational use of medicines;
- Participate in activities related to the management of health service waste, in accordance with current health legislation;
- Promote the inclusion of pharmaceutical care in Health Care Networks (HCN) and pharmaceutical services;
It is clear that the pharmacist, in the management of pharmaceutical care, identifies with a technical-scientific leadership role, thus promoting the qualification of teams, health services and social control of health;

In Brazil, the SUS has the doctrinal principles of universality, equity and integrality. It is organised on the basis of community participation and the involvement of the private sector. The SUS offers more than 40,000 basic health units, almost 6,000 hospitals and 60,000 contracted outpatient clinics, 2,500 psychosocial care centres, more than 1,000 health academies, among other facilities distributed throughout the country. Every year it provides more than 2 billion outpatient procedures and more than 11 million hospital admissions. It carries out 10 million chemotherapy and radiotherapy procedures, more than 200,000 heart surgeries and more than 150,000 vaccinations every year (data from the Ministry of Health). It develops programmes that are an international benchmark: the National Immunisation System, the HIV/AIDS Control Programme and the National Organ Transplant System, with the world's highest production of transplants carried out in public health systems. The official health system also provides the entire Brazilian population with health surveillance, food and epidemiological surveillance services, as well as universal programmes for access to medicines, among many others (MENDES, 2013; BRASIL, 2014).

Even with all this development and collective thinking, there are still shortcomings and some divergences in the way the SUS works. Naturally, given Brazil's size, health challenges, epidemiology and population reach, the system still needs to be restructured for better development.

From this perspective, the great challenge facing the SUS in contemporary society is to consolidate an integrated system that responds adequately to the population's health needs. The development of Health Care Networks (RAS), guided by Ordinance No. 4.279/2010 and Decree No. 7.508 of 28 June 2011, which regulates Organic Health Law No. 8.080 of 19 September 1990, is defined as a strategy for the operational restructuring of the health system, both in terms of its organisation and the quality and impact of the care provided on the health of the population (BRASIL, 2010; BRASIL, 2011b).

The components of the operational structure are:

Communication Centre: This is carried out by Primary/Basic Health Care, through flows and counter-flows of people, products and information between the different components of the networks (BRASIL, 2010).

Points of Care: Health care units. For example: basic health units, specialised outpatient units, haemotherapy and haematology services, psychosocial support centres, among others (BRASIL, 2010).

Diagnostic and Therapeutic Support Points: Functional units that offer support procedures such as diagnostic imaging, pathology, clinical analyses and graphic methods (BRASIL, 2010).

Support Systems: These are the institutional places in the network where services are provided that are common to all points of health care, and are transversal to the Health Care Networks. Diagnostic and Therapeutic Support Systems, Information Systems and Pharmaceutical Assistance Systems are just a few examples (BRASIL, 2010).

Logistics Systems: Where care, disease prevention and health promotion decisions are discussed. Clinical Practice Guides/Assistance Protocols are analysed, solidifying lines of care and enabling health promotion through communication between teams, services, action programmes and the standardisation of certain resources (BRASIL, 2010).

It can be seen that there are different plans for improving the system, but the integration of actions and services in the field of Pharmaceutical Assistance (PA), which is still growing slowly, is gaining prominence in favour of these improvements.

The inclusion of pharmaceutical services in the field of public policy came about with the publication of the National Medicines Policy in Brazil (BRASIL, 1998), the main observations of which are as follows:

• Ensuring the necessary safety, efficacy and quality of medicines;

• Promoting the rational use of medicines;

• The population's access to essential medicines.

The National Pharmaceutical Care Policy, formulated in 2004, provides for the necessary improvement in the care of people in health care, as well as in the use of medicines:

"A set of actions aimed at the promotion, protection and recovery of health, both individual and collective, with medicines as an essential input and with a view to access and rational use. This involves the research, development and production of medicines and supplies, as well as their selection, programming, acquisition, distribution, dispensing, guaranteeing the quality of products and services, monitoring and evaluating their use, with a view to obtaining concrete results and improving the quality of life of the population. It is also understood as a guiding public policy for the formulation of sectoral policies, including policies on medicines, science and technology, industrial development and the training of human resources, among others" (BRASIL, 2004).

Funding and the transfer of federal resources for health actions and services are passed on in the form of funding blocks. According to Ministerial Order MS/GM No. 204 of 29 January 2007, the PA block is divided into specific components such as:

a)   Basic Component, for the acquisition of medicines and pharmaceutical care supplies within the scope of Basic Health Care and those related to specific health problems and programmes, through the transfer of financial resources to municipal and/or state health departments or through the centralised acquisition of medicines by the Ministry of Health (BRASIL, 2013b).

b) Strategic Component, to finance Pharmaceutical Assistance actions for the following strategic health programmes: control of endemic diseases, such as tuberculosis, leprosy, malaria, leishmaniasis, Chagas disease and other endemic diseases of national or regional scope; antiretrovirals for the STD/AIDS programme; blood and blood products and immunobiologics, with the medicines being purchased and distributed by the Ministry of Health (BRASIL, 2010a).

c)   The Specialised Component is a strategy for access to medicines within the SUS; it is characterised by the quest to guarantee comprehensive drug treatment in outpatient settings, with special lines of care (BRASIL, 2013a).

For the rational use of medicines, a series of successful events must take place. Firstly, the therapeutic objective of using the medicine must be clearly identified; next, the appropriate medicine must be prescribed, in accordance with data on efficacy, safety and suitability for the individual. It is also necessary for the prescription to be appropriate in terms of pharmaceutical form and therapeutic regime; for the medicine to be available in a timely and accessible manner, and for it to meet the required quality criteria. It must be dispensed in appropriate ways, with guidance for the user, and the user must comply with the therapeutic regime in the best possible way, at least so that the desired therapeutic results emerge (AQUINO, 2008).

The rational use of medicines consists of using drugs correctly and only when necessary, minimising the risks of undue therapy and reducing health costs for individuals and society (MOTA et al. 2008). The efficient use of medicines requires the coordinated work of a team of professionals. The doctor, to a greater extent, selects and initiates the use of medicines, while nurses and pharmacists adjust the therapeutic plan. The former is responsible for correctly applying the dosage, while the latter ensures efficiency in interpreting and monitoring the prescribed therapy (HINDMARSH, 2001; HEPLER; SEGAL, 2003; HEPLER, 2004). Medication failures lead to economic losses, toxicity and death for patients. The role of the pharmacist ensures correct health care, promoting well-being and preventing adverse or toxicological effects (NORONHA; LIMA; MACHADO, 2008).

To ensure that the operational system and the health teams work in harmony, the SUS works on the basis of ethical and technical-operational guidelines such as (Brasil, 2014): Hierarchisation

- Primary, with more units and aimed at general practitioners;
- Secondary, intended for specialised care, and fewer in number than the primary care units;
- Tertiary, represented by teaching hospitals, fewer in number and with greater technological capacity, for difficult-to-treat cases.

The SUS hierarchisation guideline deals with exactly this: the organisation of services into levels of complexity, from basic care, established in Basic Health Units (UBS), located as close as possible to the user and prepared to organise the flow of those who need care at other levels, through medical or specialised care, to high complexity, aimed at situations that require highly specialised technological resources. There is also emergency care. This structure aims to improve the programming and planning of the system's actions and services. It is not always necessary for a municipality to have all levels of health care installed in its territory in order to guarantee comprehensive care for its population. Particularly in the case of small municipalities, this can be done through regional pacts that guarantee their populations access to all levels of complexity in the system. The priority for all municipalities is to have basic care operating in full and effective conditions. (BRASIL, 2009, P.41)

Hierarchisation seeks, among other things, economies of scale and thus greater possibilities of guaranteeing compliance with ethical principles.

Regionalisation

It is the application of the principle of territoriality, i.e. the democracy of spaces and responsibilities. The management of health services must be organised in such a way that the entire population is included in territories covered, at the very least, by basic care and referred to health units at other, more complex levels.

Delimiting territories and establishing responsibilities allows the population to be known and their needs to be met, in accordance with the principle of universality, prioritising those most in need (equity) and in a comprehensive manner. Regionalisation should guide the decentralisation of health actions and services, identifying and setting up health regions - territorial spaces in which health care actions will be developed, with the aim of achieving greater resoluteness and quality in results, as well as greater capacity for rational management.

Popular participation

This principle guarantees the participation of the population in the construction of public health policies and in the management of the SUS, at all municipal, state and federal levels, via Health Councils and Conferences.

There is a health care model such as the Family Health Strategy (ESF), adopted by the Ministry of Health. The actions of the ESF are aimed at:

- Expanding coverage and improving the quality of care;
- Organising access to the system;
- Comprehensive care;
- Raising public awareness of the main local diseases and their determinants;
- Encouraging public participation in the control of the health system.

Pharmacists are still little in demand to integrate SUS care processes, partly because of the high demand for their services in pharmaceutical care management processes, but also because of the lack of tradition among professionals themselves in occupying this space, despite the commitment of many already devoted to it, particularly since the last decade.

The pharmacist's participation in care processes must be based on their interaction with users and the community, and does not depend solely on having the medicine as an instrument of intervention: the pharmacist's role in assisting users and the community goes beyond the medicine; it encompasses health care in its broadest sense.

Living conditions, access to goods and services, education, work, political and social emancipation can and should be part of the pharmacist's work.

REFERENCES

BRAZIL. Ministry of Health. Ordinance No. 2.488, of 21 October 2011. Approves the National Primary Care Policy, establishing revised guidelines and norms for the organisation of Primary Care, for the Family Health Strategy (ESF) and the Community Health Agents Programme (PACS). Diario Oficial da Uniao, Poder Executive, Brasilia/DF, 24 Oct 2011a. Section 1, p. 48. Available at: . Accessed on: 5 October 2014.

MENDES, E. V. Health care networks. 2. ed. Brasilia: Pan American Health Organisation, 2011. 549 p.

MENDES, E. V. Health care networks. Ciencia & Saude Coletiva, [S.l.], v. 15, n. 5, p. 2297-2305, 2010.

MENDES, E. V. 25 years of the Unified Health System: results and challenges. Estudos avan^ados, [S.l.], v. 27, n. 78, p. 27-34, 2013. Available at: . Accessed on: 15 Sep. 2014.

SANTOS, N. R. Sistema Unico de Saude - 2010: space for a turning point. O mundo da saude, Sao Paulo, v. 34, n. 1, p. 8-19, 2010.

COSTA, K. S.; NASCIMENTO JR., J. M. HORUS: technological innovation in pharmaceutical care in the Unified Health System. Revista de Saude Publica, [S.l.], v. 46, supl. 1, p. 91-99, dec. 2012.

COSTA, K. S.; FRANCISCO, P. M. S. B.; BARROS, M. B. A. Knowledge and Use of the Brazilian Popular Pharmacy Programme: a population-based study in the municipality of Campinas/SP. Epidemiol. Serv. Saude, Brasilia, v. 23, n. 3, p. 397-408, jul./set. 2014.

AQUINO, D. S. Why should the rational use of medicines be a priority? Ciencia & Saude Coletiva, [S.l.], v. 13, n. p. 733-736, 2008.

MOTA, D. M. et al. Rational use of medicines: an economic approach for decision-making. Ciencia & Saude Coletiva, [S.l.], v. 13, p. 589-601, 2008.

HINDMARSH, K. W. Optimal drug therapy: the role of the pharmacist in bridging the gap between knowledge and action. - e Canadian Journal of Clinical Pharmacology, [S.l.], v. 8, n. 2, p. 53A-54A, 2001. Suppl. A.

NORONHA, J.C.; LIMA, L.D.; MACHADO,C.V. O Sistema Unico de Saude - SUS. In: GIOVANELLA, L. ET AL.(org.). Politicas e sistemas de saude no Brasil. Rio de Janeiro: Fiocruz, 2008.

Chapter 6

THE IMPORTANCE OF CLINICAL PHARMACIST INTERVENTIONS IN DIFFERENT HOSPITAL SETTINGS

Thays de Lima Ferreira[1] ; Michelle Melgarejo da Rosa[2]

1 - Pharmacy student at UniFBV Wyden University Centre

2 - Professor of Pharmacy at UniFBV Wyden University Centre

Clinical Pharmacy is an area of activity for pharmacists in hospitals, which has Resolution No. 585 of 29 August 2013, which regulates the clinical attributions of pharmacists, reporting the rights and duties of this professional. The term "Clinical Pharmacy" became popular in the 1960s as a result of the indiscriminate use of thalidomide, which led pharmacists to realise the importance of providing assistance to users and not just manipulation and industrial production (Pereira and Freitas, 2008). Thalidomide, an anti-inflammatory, sedative and hypnotic drug, became known for inducing foetal malformation, being teratogenic and therefore currently contraindicated for pregnant women. From this history, pharmacoepidemiology and pharmacovigilance began in order to provide better quality assurance for patients. At this time in Brazil, pharmacists worked in areas such as clinical analyses, industry and the food sector.

The picture began to change in the 1970s and 1980s when pharmacists at teaching hospitals began to introduce unit doses and clinical activities (CRF) into their work routine. In these same decades, the subjects of clinical pharmacy, hospital pharmacy and pharmacotherapy began to appear on university pharmacy programmes, giving rise to clinical activities outside hospitals as well. In 1993, the International Pharmaceutical Federation (FIP), held in Tokyo, amended the document "Good Pharmacy Practice: Quality Standards for Pharmaceutical Services", supported by the WHO. This document emphasises that "the mission of pharmacy practice is to dispense medicines and other health care products and services, helping people and society to use them in the best possible way". This means that the role of the clinical pharmacist is to maintain patient safety and quality of life, reduce and prevent problems for the individual by analysing prescriptions together with the multidisciplinary team, and reduce the hospital's mortality rate, reducing the patient's length of stay, speeding up their improvement, making sure that the patient understands the treatment, the timetable and the adverse effects that the medication can cause, making sure that the medication is used rationally and not leaving the patient with any doubts about the pharmacotherapy. The pharmacist can also plan the therapy according to the particularities of each patient, in order to reduce the adverse effects of the drug (CFF). These activities contribute to hospital pharmacoeconomics by reducing hospital costs and improving patient care.

The aim here is to show how the intervention of the clinical pharmacist generates satisfactory results for all those involved in the treatment (patient, family, multidisciplinary team and the hospital).

The Role of the Clinical Pharmacist in the First Aid Unit (UPA)

The UPA is a sector of the hospital that receives people in emergency situations, who may or may not be at risk of death and need emergency care. Few hospitals have clinical pharmacists working in the UPA. A data collection carried out at the First Aid Unit in Morumbi at the Hospital Israelita Albert Einsten in 2010 demonstrated the importance of the Clinical Pharmacy Service in this sector, through the number of interventions carried out, with a total of 3542 medical prescriptions that had 1238 pharmaceutical interventions, together with the interdisciplinary team. In this data collection, 17 types of pharmaceutical intervention were carried out to benefit the treatment and the patient.

The five that had the highest incidence were: prescriptions that had an unusual dose, inappropriate dilution of medication, unusual route of administration, inappropriate infusion time and inappropriate frequency of administration.

With this study, we can see the different interventions that the clinical pharmacist can carry out and how these can favour the best prognosis of therapies, helping the hospital to run more smoothly.

The pharmacist is the right person to find out if the prescription is unsuitable for administration to the patient, if the drug is diluted, if the way the drug is administered is unsuitable, if the drugs are incompatible, if the dose is higher or lower than necessary, and if there are any other interventions that are appropriate for optimising drug therapy and patient safety.

The rational use of the drug, the prevention of adverse effects and the guarantee of a reduction in costs for the hospital.

It's important to emphasise that patient contact is also a function of the pharmacy clinic. This professional aims to gather information about patients and use it intelligently in favour of their well-being. As well as providing therapeutic support to the patient, this professional must explain possible adverse effects of therapies and how to minimise them to the patient and their family. The clinical pharmacist is an important person responsible for transmitting hospital information, both at the bedside and through health actions and research (Miranda et al., 2011).

The Role of the Clinical Pharmacist with a Focus on the Elderly

Greater attention should be paid to elderly patients, as they are usually polymedicated. They have a slower metabolism and a modified physiological system that can lead to pharmacokinetic and pharmacodynamic problems with drugs, and they are also a margin of the population common to chronic non-communicable diseases such as hypertension and diabetes (Viana et al., 2017). In view of this, contact between the patient and the pharmacist becomes extremely important in order to promote rational therapy, free of drug-related problems (DRPs) and adverse drug reactions (ADRs), reducing toxicity and increasing user comfort. Always taking into account the particularities of the user in order to achieve better results and improve quality of life.

In 2015, data was collected at the Intermediate Care Unit of the Hospital das Clinicas of the Faculty of Medicine of the University of Sao Paulo, in which 386 prescriptions were evaluated, including 212 pharmaceutical interventions. 64.3% of these interventions were accepted and had a change in the prescription, 28.5% were not accepted and 7.2% were verbally accepted but had no change in the prescription. The accepted interventions that had changes to the prescription were carried out in person with the medical and nursing team in order to define the best course of action to be followed according to the patient's needs. However, the interventions that were not accepted show that the clinical experience still needs to be improved in order to bring it closer together and provide more precise interventions. The rates of interventions that were accepted verbally but had no change in the prescription were due to the patient's rapid progression to death, leaving no time to change the prescription. This data was also due to some patients being transferred to another clinic. The pharmacist in this hospital setting provides better monitoring of the patient's clinical situation through the analysis of medical prescriptions, proving that the pharmacist effectively contributes to the multiprofessional role with a focus on elderly patients, through the high percentage of interventions carried out in this study.

The role of the clinical pharmacist in the discharge of transplant patients After transplants, it is necessary for the patient to adapt to new care. Changes in diet, use of medication, becoming a polymedicated patient, frequent examinations are some examples of these changes (Lima et al., 2016). The clinical pharmacist, together with the multi-professional team, will help the patient in this new post-transplant reality. The pharmacist's role is to make the patient realise that they are responsible for their own treatment, guiding them and planning their medication according to the reality and particularities of the individual. Once again, the pharmacist must analyse the prescription in order to prevent, detect and resolve problems related to the therapy. In a study carried out at the Renal and Hepatic Transplant Unit of the Walter Cantidio University Hospital in Fortaleza - CE, the clinical pharmacist's interventions were analysed from January to July 2014. During this period, 74 hospital discharges were analysed and 59 of them had PRMs, 67.8% of which were related to the non-prescription of necessary medication, 10.1% to errors in the dose of medication (under- or over-dosing), 6.8% to the absence of a request for an examination, and 5.1% to missing or inadequate documentation for the dispensation of medication. The pharmaceutical interventions presented in this study were classified as preventive and appropriate, as they prevented worsening of the clinical condition and improved the quality of care and reduced patient toxicity. Thus, it was proven that pharmaceutical intervention prevents negative results associated with pharmacotherapy and that the pharmacist, in addition to advising the patient about the new treatment, should also be present at the time of prescription together with the doctor, to ensure that all the necessary pharmacotherapy is present and to analyse the patient's tests to prevent possible PRMs.

The significant number of interventions accepted by the healthcare team reinforces the role that the clinical pharmacist has to play in the interdisciplinary team, since pharmacotherapeutic monitoring promotes better control of the patient's pathology, due to the patient's better knowledge of the medication and better communication with the healthcare team (Pereira and Freitas, 2008). These indicators contribute to reducing medication errors, adverse reactions, prevention and early detection of diseases and unnecessary costs to the health system (Viana et al., 2017; Miranda et al., 2011). Although clinical pharmacy is an area that is still developing, these activities publicise the importance of the work of the professional pharmacist, who is gradually becoming an essential part of the various hospital settings.

REFERENCES:

Pereira, Leonardo Regis Leira; Freitas, Osvlado de. **The evolution of Pharmaceutical Care and the outlook for Brazil**. Revista Brasileira de Ciencias Farmaceuticas Brazilian Journal of Pharmaceutical Sciences vol. 44, n. 4, Oct./Dec., 2008.

Martins, Bruna Cristina Cardoso et al. **Pharmaceutical Care for Transplant Patients in a University Hospital: Pharmaceutical Interventions Carried Out. Walter Cantidio University Hospital (HUWC) Federal University of Ceara**. Fortaleza (CE), 2011.

Federal Pharmacy Council of the State of Sao Paulo. **Clinical Pharmacy in the World: Pharmacies in Europe and South America stand out for differentiated services and integration with the health system.** Revista do Farmaceutico n.129 February-Mar^o-April, 2017.

Bromati, Ana Carla; Fontes, Profa Dr Cassiana Mendes Bertoncello. **Manual for pharmaceutical care for informal carers of the elderly.** Universidade Estadual Paulista Julio de Mesquita Filho Faculdade de Medicina de Botucatu Multiprofessional Residency Programme in Adult and Elderly Health, 2018.

Federal Pharmacy Council. Pioneer in the field talks about the importance of pharmacists working in hospitals. Available: http://crfms.org.br/noticias/farmaceutico/3911-pioneiro-na- area-fala-obre-importancia-da-atuacao-do-farmaceutico-em-hospitais, 2017.

Viana, Stephanie de Souza Costa et al. **Interventions of the clinical pharmacist in an Intermediate Care Unit for elderly patients**. Hospital das Clinicas, Faculty of Medicine, University of Sao Paulo, Sao Paulo, 2017.

Miranda, Talita Muniz Maloni et al. **Interventions performed by the clinical pharmacist in the emergency department.** Hospital Israelita Albert Einstein - HIAE, Sao Paulo (SP),Brazil, 2011.

Lima. Livia Falcao et al. **Pharmaceutical guidance at hospital discharge for transplant patients: a strategy for patient safety.** Walter Cantidio University Hospital, Federal University of Ceara, Fortaleza, CE, Brazil, 2016.

COLUMNIST PORTAL EDUCAO. The emergence of pharmaceutical chemistry   .
Available   at:https://www.portaleducacao.com.br/conteudo/artigos/farmacia/o-surgimento-da-farmacia-clinica/21017

Federal Pharmacy Council. Regulates the clinical attributions of pharmacists and makes other provisions. Resolution no. 585 of 29 August 2013. Available: http://www.cff.org.br/userfiles/file/resolucoes/585.pdf.

Chapter 7

THE PHARMACIST'S ROLE IN PREVENTING MEDICATION ERRORS

Layla Lais Ribeiro Fragoso[1] , Amanda Emanuela da Silva Rocha Melo[1] , Michelle Melgarejo da Rosa[2]

1 - Pharmacy student at UniFBV Wyden University Centre
2 - Professor of Pharmacy at UniFBV Wyden University Centre

Medication errors are one of the biggest causes of death in hospitals. In order to reduce these cases, multidisciplinary teams have been set up in which pharmacists play a fundamental role in providing assistance, assessing prescriptions and controlling the dispensing of medicines. This type of collaboration between pharmacists reduces the risks of drug interactions, high doses and toxic effects for patients, among other errors. In this chapter, we'll look at the pharmacist's contributions to the multidisciplinary team and their role in hospital pharmacy to reduce errors.

PHARMACEUTICAL ASSISTANCE

Initially, the focus of pharmacists in healthcare was more on improving financial resources, management and logistics. However, there was a need to broaden the areas of activity, aiming for general health care, working together with the multidisciplinary team within the hospital.
Resolution No. 338 of 6 May 2004 mentions the expanded role of the pharmacist in pharmaceutical care:
"Pharmaceutical assistance is a set of actions aimed at promoting, protecting and recovering health, both individual and collective, with medicines as an essential input and with a view to access and rational use. This involves research, development and production of medicines and supplies, as well as their selection, programming, acquisition, distribution, dispensing, quality assurance and services. Pharmacists must monitor and evaluate their use, with a view to obtaining concrete results and improving the quality of life of the population.
It is a model of pharmaceutical practice, developed in the context of Pharmaceutical Care and comprising attitudes, ethical values, behaviours, skills, commitments and co-responsibilities in the prevention of diseases, promotion and recovery of health, in an integrated way with the health team. It is the pharmacist's direct interaction with the user, aimed at rational pharmacotherapy and obtaining defined and measurable results aimed at improving quality of life. This interaction must also involve the conceptions of its subjects, respecting their bio-psycho-social specificities, from the point of view

of the integrality of health actions".

The resolution makes explicit the importance of the pharmacist in the therapeutic sphere, in caring for the patient in the recovery and protection of health, without discarding the rational use of medicines that will be promoted by the pharmacist's action within the hospital area.

PHARMACEUTICAL CARE CYCLE

The pharmaceutical care cycle involves six essential stages for the flow of medicines in hospitals: selection, programming, acquisition, storage, distribution and dispensing (Cavallini and Bisson, 2010).

SELECTION, PROGRAMMING AND ACQUISITION

The selection of medicines and supplies is important for evaluating new developments in the industry and improving therapies. It also evaluates the safety, efficacy and cost-effectiveness of different therapies. Areas that work together in these processes include pharmacoepidemiology, pharmacoeconomics, pharmacovigilance and clinical and therapeutic pharmacology.

The programme analyses the target region to meet the needs of the population, planning quantities and adjusting them to the Average Monthly Consumption (AMC), epidemiological profile, historical consumption and supply of services.

STORAGE AND DISTRIBUTION

Storage is responsible for ensuring the quality of medicines with the correct storage required for each one. It must follow the standards stipulated by the institution. Care must be taken from the moment the medicines enter the hospital until the stock is organised. Organisation, in turn, is very important, as it arranges the medicines in such a way that they are perfectly identified and structured. In this way, dispensing errors can be prevented.

Distribution is the stage where medicines leave storage and are sent to other sectors. All the information on incoming and outgoing batches must be correctly computerised.

DISPENSATION

Dispensing is the stage most relevant to the subject. This involves the pharmacist's role in preventing medication errors.

At this stage, greater attention is paid to ensuring that the medicines are sent to the correct patient, the effectiveness of the information on use is emphasised, and the correct packaging is checked so as not to alter the quality of the medicine. Naturally, the medicine must be labelled correctly (Malaoli, 2009).

During dispensing, the pharmacist can detect small errors in dosage, incorrect medication, incorrect prescribed route, and if there isn't an excessive amount of medication being administered. This is why analysing the prescription is an integral part of the pharmacist's role in health care.

ANALYSING MEDICAL PRESCRIPTIONS

Analysing prescriptions prevents medication errors, such as wrong doses for the age and weight of patients, drug interactions, drugs that have pharmacokinetics that can harm an already weakened organ, administration by the wrong route, administration of the dose at the wrong time, as well as the physical and emotional state of the professional, which can lead to errors, even due to excessive working hours. It is the pharmacist's role to suggest improved therapy, reducing the number of drugs prescribed and, consequently, pharmacological interactions. The pharmacist is the professional responsible for the drugs and their correct use. Multidisciplinary work aims to improve the health system and ensure therapeutic and clinical stability. Even though this routine is not yet dominant, different plans and ways are being sought to make pharmacist-doctor work increasingly necessary and effective. Greater recognition of the latter could change the way health care is provided (Finatto and Caon, 2015).

Anvisa has issued a resolution that the pharmacist must assess the medical prescription in terms of its viability, stability and the physico-chemical compatibility of the components. This is where oncology drug prescriptions are being targeted.

MEDICATION ERRORS IN THE ONCOLOGICAL SECTOR The mistaken administration of high doses of some cytostatics results in serious toxicity and the death of patients. Non-conformities in prescriptions to oncology patients can be catastrophic due to the narrow therapeutic margin of antineoplastic drugs. Preventing medication errors is one of the priorities in improving the pharmacotherapy process for oncology patients (Oliboni, 2009).

The National Health Surveillance Agency, in a Resolution issued in 2004, states that the person responsible for preparing antineoplastic therapy is the pharmacist. In addition to assessing the medical prescription with regard to the viability, stability and physical-chemical compatibility of the components with each other, he must examine its suitability for the protocols established by the multidisciplinary antineoplastic therapy team and the legibility and identification of the registration with the Regional Medical Council (CRM).

MEDICATION ERRORS IN CHEMOTHERAPY

Serious consequences such as deafness, kidney failure, persistent aplasia or even death have been reported in the literature. Errors in drug selection are often not realised by pharmacists because the prescription often does not provide the adequate information needed to determine the suitability of a particular therapy.

STRATEGIES FOR REDUCING MEDICATION ERRORS

- Standardisation of processes and effective action by the Pharmacy and Therapeutics Commission (CFT);
- Written protocols and a checklist of routines and processes;
- Constant training and access to information for the health team;
- Reduce improvisation and work shift changes;
- Encourage the automation of processes with the entire healthcare team, especially prescribers.

The role of the pharmacist is fundamental in minimising harmful errors to the patient. Their duties and responsibilities allow them to intervene in both the administrative and clinical spheres, making them very important in guiding and implementing processes that can improve patient services and prevent errors.

REFERENCES:

Cavallini ME, Bisson MP. **Farmacia hospitalar enfoque em sistemas de saude.** 2 ed. Barueri: Editora Manole, 2010.

Oliboni LS, Camargo AL. **Validation of the oncology prescription: the pharmacist's role in preventing medication errors**. Rev HCPA 2009.

National Health Surveillance Agency. Resolution RDC no. 220, of 21 September 2004. **Approves the technical regulations for the operation of antineoplastic therapy services.** Official Gazette of the Union. Brasilia, DF, 2004.

Leape LL, Bates DW, Cullen DJ. **Systems analysis of adverse drug events.** JAMA. 1995.

Fernandez MJH, Baena-Canada JM, Bautista MJM, Arellano EA, Palacios MVG. **Impact of computerised chemotherapy prescriptions on the prevention of medication errors.** Clin Transl Oncol. 2006;8(11):821-25.

Ministry of Health, National Health Surveillance Agency. Disponivel em:

>http://portal.anvisa.gov.br/documents/10181/2718376/RDC_67_2007_COMP.pdf/5de28862   -
e018-4287-892e-a2add589ac26<. Accessed on: 24 Nov. 2018.

Rego MM, Comarella L. **The role of pharmaceutical analysis of hospital prescriptions. Caderno saude e desenvolvimento.** Vol.7 n.4 - 2015.

Finatto RB, Caon S. **Analysis of "near misses" in the prescription process detected by the clinical pharmacist.** Ver. Bras. Farm. 96(1): 1042- 1054, 2015.

Malaoli BG. **Pharmacotherapeutic manual for improving hospital pharmacy practices.** Belo Horizonte: UFMG, 2009.

Chapter 8
ALZHEIMER'S DISEASE IN THE CONTEXT OF HOSPITAL PHARMACY

Glauciane Valeska da Silva[1] ; Rayane da Silva Morais[1] ; Michelle Melgarejo da Rosa[2]

1 - Pharmacy student at UniFBV Wyden University Centre
2 - Professor of Pharmacy at UniFBV Wyden University Centre

Alzheimer's disease (AD) was first described in 1906 by Dr Alois Alzheimer when he published a case study of one of his patients called August D., aged 51. Initially, Auguste constantly accused her husband of infidelity for no apparent justifiable reason. Shortly afterwards, she began to show memory deficits, disorientation and, at times, would scream loudly because she believed that someone might hurt her or take her life. The symptoms of cognitive impairment became increasingly intense. August died four years after the first symptoms appeared. When Alois studied August's brain, he noticed that there was death of neuronal cells in the cortex region (an area related to cognition) as well as altered cells that formed a tangle of neurofibrils composed of tau proteins and senile plaques formed by the beta-amyloid protein. These neurofibrils and senile plaques were responsible for the death of neurons and the reduction of neuronal synapses (INSTITUTO ALZHEIMER BRASIL, 2018).

AD is considered to be an irreversible and progressive neurodegenerative disease that causes the death of neurons, thus compromising certain functions of the central nervous system. Initially, the disease damages the hippocampus, affecting short-term memory, and later compromises associative cortical areas. According to the World Health Organisation (WHO, 2013), the hallmark of AD is a progressive decline in memory, reasoning, understanding, the ability to calculate, learn and perform common everyday tasks. Other symptoms include speech difficulties, personality changes and language comprehension, including progressive impairment of daily activities and other changes that compromise quality of life (LOPES and GORINI SILVA, 2006; FALCO et al. 2012; CORREIA et al., 2015; BIGUETI et al., 2018). The disease is caused by a lack of synapses in the hippocampus, entorhinal cortex, cerebral cortex and ventral striatum, areas responsible for cognitive functions. In these regions, AD sufferers have fibrillar reservoirs located in the walls of blood vessels together with a variety of different senile plaques, composed of the beta-amyloid protein which generates the accumulation of abnormal filaments of the tau protein and, as a consequence, the formation of neurofibrillary tangles (NFT). These alterations culminate in the stimulation of glial cells, which are responsible for the central inflammatory response, increasing neuronal inflammation and leading to neural loss (SERENIKI et al.., 2008; BIGUETI et al., 2018).

AD can be classified into: initial, intermediate, advanced or terminal stages. In the early stages, manifestations are superficial and include speech difficulties, significant memory loss, lack of initiative and motivation in previously pleasurable activities, signs of depression and aggression (GRAHAM et al., 2000). In the middle stages, there may be a loss of speech ability, making it impossible to name simple objects, as well as difficulty in executing movements.

In the terminal stages, extreme sleep difficulties, behavioural changes of irritability and aggression; psychotic symptoms; inability to walk, talk and carry out personal care (RAMOS apud GALLUCCI NETO; TAMELINI; FORLENZA, 2005).

According to LOPES and collaborators quoted by MARINHO in 1997, "AD affects approximately 4% of people aged between 65 and 75, 10% of those aged between 75 and 85 and 17% of all people over 85". The likelihood of developing Alzheimer's is therefore proportional to age. However, it can also occur in neurologically normal individuals (GOODMAN and GILMAN, 2012).

According to the 2015 report by the Alzheimer's Disease International Association (ADI), it is estimated that there are around 46.8 million people in the world with the disease, and that this figure could reach 74.7 million by 2030 and 131.5 million by 2050. According to the report, currently a case of dementia is detected every 3.2 seconds and by 2050 there will be a new case every second (INSTITUTO ALZHEIMER BRASIL, 2018).

With the increase in life expectancy, the prevalence of the disease has become higher, especially in developed countries (FERNANDES et al., 2017).

Hospital pharmacists play an important role in the prognosis and treatment of Alzheimer's and other neurodegenerative diseases. Since this professional is responsible for providing pharmaceutical care to family members and patients, whether at their bedside or not, explaining what it is, how the pathogenesis occurs, and what treatments are needed. Some studies have shown that patients who were given information about what was happening in their therapy had better adherence to their medication and consequently an improvement in their current clinical state. The hospital pharmacist also observes and verifies that the prescription is correct, analysing whether there are possible pharmacological and food interactions, and whether the dose and route of administration are appropriate. In this way, there has been a reduction in medical errors and an improvement in therapeutic adherence (TRINDADE, 2017).

Etiopathology

The precursor protein B-amyloid is highly relevant to the genesis of senile plaques formed between neurons. The tau protein, which makes up the neurofibrillary tangles, is also characteristic of the condition, but there is still no knowledge of its relationship with senile plaques. As for genetics, it is known that the e(4) allele of the apolipoprotein E (ApoE) gene is around 3 times more frequent in people with AD and that people who are homozygous for the gene are at greater risk of the disease than those who are not homozygous (WHO apud W, 1997; SELKOE 1997).

Apolipoprotein E (apoE) is undoubtedly an important risk factor for AD. Individuals homozygous for the apoE4 allele have a higher risk of developing AD at any stage of life than individuals homozygous for the apoE2 allele. The mechanism by which apoE4 increases the chances of developing AD has not yet been fully clarified, but it is believed to produce alterations in the aggregation or processing of P-amyloid (AP) (GOODMAN & GILMAN apud MARLEY et al., 2006).

According to Goodman & Gilman (2012, p. 610 apud SELKOE & PODLINSY, 2002) "AD does not have a defined hereditary pattern, but mutations in genes that code for the amyloid precursor protein (APP) and pressenilin proteins involved in the processing of APP, cause hereditary forms of the disease. According to Falco et al (2016), there are three hypotheses for the development of AD. These include: The cholinergic hypothesis, the glutamatergic hypothesis and the amyloid cascade hypothesis. In the cholinergic hypothesis, a reduction in the enzyme choline acetyltransferase, which is responsible for synthesising acetylcholine in the cortex and hippocampus, causes a reduction in the concentration of acetylcholine (ACh) in these regions and this reduction leads to the death of cholinergic neurons due to inactivity. As ACh plays a major role in learning and memory, it is believed that this deficit in ACH production may favour the development of AD. In the glutamatergic hypothesis, certain conducts, such as alterations in the cell's energy metabolism, can trigger hyperstimulation of glutamatergic receptors (NMDA), which in turn deregulate intracellular Ca^{2+} levels, triggering neuronal death by hyperstimulation. In the amyloid cascade hypothesis, AD symptoms are associated with various neuronal and extracellular lesions in the limbic and cerebral cortex. Another characteristic of this hypothesis is the existence of plaques, also known as senile plaques, formed by beta-amyloid peptide. These injuries lead to neuronal death due to oxidative stress and/or inflammation, causing a reduction in the size of the cortex which, in turn, atrophies due to local neuronal inactivity, reducing in size and increasing interneuronal spaces (PRADO apud PRATICO D 2002; HOOZEMANS J. 2003; CALLAHAN C 1995).

Genetics

The genes currently known to be associated with AD are: amyloid precursor protein (APP), presenilin 1 (PSEN1), presenilin 2 (PSEN2). Mutations in APP are responsible for 5% of hereditary AD. PSEN1 mutations are responsible for most cases of hereditary AD, while PSEN2 mutations are the rarest (ABN Manual recommendations in ALZHEIMER apud GOATE A, ET AL 1991; SHERRINGTON R, ET AL 1995; LEVY-LAHAD E, ET AL 1995; WATTAMWAR PR, ET AL 2010; WATTAMWAR PR,

2005).

Some studies show that there is no way of intervening when it comes to genetic factors, but lifestyle habits can either delay or accelerate the development of AD. Among the causes that can be intervened upon is the maintenance of healthy lifestyle habits that include adequate nutrition, regular physical exercise and adequate rest. These factors are fundamental for avoiding the development of pathologies such as cardiovascular disorders, cerebrovascular diseases such as cerebral thrombosis, dyslipidemia, diabetes and metabolic syndromes (PRADO apud PATTERSON C. et al, 2007).

Pathophysiology

AD sufferers present amyloid plaques in the medial temporal lobe, erythrocyte cortex and hippocampus, formed by the accumulation of P-amyloid protein and microtubule-associated tau protein tangles. It is currently believed that the accumulation of P-amyloid proteins is the initial factor, which leads to a deregulation of the tau protein, resulting in cell dysfunction and neuronal death (GOODMAN & GILMAN 2012, page 619).

According to Goodman & Gilman (2012, p. 619), the signs and symptoms are attributed to dysfunctions in these brain regions, which cause temporary loss of previous memory, repetitive questions, placing objects in inappropriate places, missing appointments and forgetting everyday details, as well as memory deficit. When they don't limit common functions, they are classified as mild cognitive impairment (MCI). These symptoms progress until they affect other regions of the brain.

Neurochemistry

The main disorder in AD is a decrease in the neurotransmitter acetylcholine (ACh). This absence leads to atrophy and degeneration of cholinergic neurons, especially those located in the basal forebrain. In addition, certain cholinergic antagonists can also cause a state of mental confusion similar to that of AD. These factors have led to the cholinergic hypothesis, where ACh deficiency is the key factor in triggering the disease (GOODMAN & GILMAN apud, PERRY, 1986).

Treatment

There is currently no treatment capable of preventing the progression of AD. What is done is to alleviate the symptoms (RAMOS, 2017)

Treatment of cognitive symptoms

The drugs used are: Donepezil, rivastigmine, galantamine and tacrine. These belong to the group of reversible inhibitors of the enzyme acetylcholinesterase (AChE). AChE is responsible for the degradation of ACh in the synaptic cleft. Once the enzyme is inhibited, ACh remains active for longer in the synaptic cleft. Tacrine and rivastigmine have an inhibitory action on butyrylcholinesterase, which can cause peripheral side effects. However, AChE inhibitors are the first choice for treating cognitive deficits in mild to moderate AD (PRADO, 2010).

Treatment of behavioural symptoms

Behavioural symptoms include irritability, agitation, paranoia, depression and anxiety. These symptoms are responsible for patients being hospitalised. It should be noted that treatment can be difficult and that non-pharmacological therapies such as cognitive rehabilitation/reinforcement/training, psychoeducational programmes and training for carers, physical activity, other occupational therapy strategies, music therapy, physiotherapy and speech therapy should be used before the use of drugs (ABN RECOMMENDATIONS MANUAL ON ALZHEIMER'S, 2011).

In the treatment of behavioural symptoms, atypical antipsychotic drugs such as risperidone, olanzapine and quetiapine are effective in controlling agitation and psychosis. However, risperidone and olanzapine are restricted due to their adverse effects (GOODMAN & GILMAN, 2012 page 622).

Diagnosis

The diagnosis of AD is often delayed due to the fact that the symptoms of the disease are similar to those common to age. For this reason, the patient's clinical history must be taken into account, together with laboratory and neuroimaging tests that allow the patient to be diagnosed while still alive. As the disease progresses, the symptoms of AD become increasingly severe and clear and the diagnosis more obvious (BIGUETI apud ASSOCIA^AO BRASILEIRA ALZHEIMER, 2012). The definitive diagnosis of AD can only be made by analysing *post-mortem* brain tissue (XIMENES, 2014).

The use of markers makes it possible to detect B-amyloid peptide and tau protein, either in lower concentrations in the cerebrospinal fluid or by identifying deposits of this peptide in the brain, using new molecular neuroimaging methods such as positron emission tomography. When these alterations occur and neuronal damage is associated with them, the diagnosis can be made with certainty. However, this form of diagnosis cannot yet be considered routine due to the lack of standardisation and is restricted to research use only (ABN RECOMMENDATIONS MANUAL ON ALZHEIMER'S, 2011).

Also according to the ABN Manual of Recommendations on Alzheimer's, the basic clinical criteria for diagnosis include:

- Dementia: Cognitive or behavioural symptoms that interfere with routine activities; Decreased reasoning and performance; Mental confusion.
- Cognitive impairment through the patient's anamnesis and neuropsychological assessment of the patient's mental state.
- Cognitive impairment includes Loss of memory, without the possibility of retrieving and/or retaining information; Lack of ability to reason and understand situations of risk or danger;
- Difficulty recognising common people, places and objects.
- Communication difficulties (reading, understanding, expressing and writing)
Behavioural changes such as sudden mood swings (agitation, disinterest, social isolation, obsessive or compulsive)

Complementary tests

Laboratory

To this day, there is no biological or serological marker available for detecting or monitoring AD, because TAU protein concentrates are difficult to detect. Concentrations of B-amyloid peptides are unreliable because their results are varied and contradictory. As there is no evidence that this peptide is reduced in AD, this parameter cannot be used to aid diagnosis. Laboratory tests that can help with the diagnosis are: complete blood count, serum creatinine concentrations, TSH, albumin, liver enzymes, vitamin B12, folic acid, calcium, serological reactions for syphilis and, in patients under the age of 60 with atypical clinical presentations or suggestive symptoms, HIV serology should be used to investigate potential secondary causes of dementia syndrome (ABN RECOMMENDATIONS MANUAL ON ALZHEIMER'S, 2011). Image

Computerised tomography (CT) and magnetic resonance imaging (MRI) of the brain are used in the initial assessment. MRI is the most effective method for detecting changes and is the method of choice (ABN RECOMMENDATIONS MANUAL ON ALZHEIMER'S, 2011).

Statistically, the number of cases of AD will almost double in 10 years. Even with the use of non-pharmacological therapies, AD treatment is still based on drugs such as donepezil, rivastigmine, galantamine and tacrine, which are the first choice because they inhibit the reuptake of ACh, leading to improved cognition. However, they generate a number of adverse effects, which require intense monitoring. The same happens with the use of antipsychotics which control agitation and psychosis, but their use is rarely indicated due to adverse effects. In this way, pharmacists play an extremely important role, as they are responsible for monitoring the patient's response to medication, monitoring the progression of the disease and playing a fundamental role in ensuring adherence to treatment by advising family members, carers and patients about the pathology and the adverse

53

effects that can occur during treatment.

References

BIGUET, B. C. P. ; LELLIS, J. Z. ; DIAS, J. C. R. **ESSENTIAL NUTRIENTS IN THE PREVENTION OF ALZHEIMER'S DISEASE,** Bebedouro - SP, Revista Ciencias Nutricionais Online, v.2, n.2, p.18-25, 2018.

BRAZIL. SAS/WHO Ordinance No. 1.298. **CLINICAL PROTOCOL AND THERAPEUTIC GUIDELINES ALZHEIMER'S DISEASE**, p. 147 - 167, 2013.

DEMENTIA & NEUROPSYCHOLOGIA, **RECOMENDACOES IN ALZHEIMER,** Sao Paulo - SP, v. 5, p. 5 - 48, 2011.

FALCO, A. et al. **ALZHEIMER'S DISEASE: ETIOLOGICAL HYPOTHESIS AND TREATMENT PERSPECTIVES,** Rio de Janeiro - RJ. Chem. Nova, Vol. 39, No. 1, p. 63-80, 2016.

FERNANDES J. S. G. ; ANDRADE M. S. **REVIEW OF ALZHEIMER'S DISEASE: DIAGNOSIS, EVOLUTION AND CARE,** Osasco - SP. PSYCHOLOGY, HEALTH & DISEASES, Vol. 75(1), p. 131-140, 2017.

GOODMAN & GILMAN. **THE PHARMACOLOGICAL BASES OF THERAPEUTICS**, 12. Ed, Porto Alegre - RS, McGraw-Hill, 2012.

ALZHEIMER INSTITUTE BRAZIL.

LEITE, J. C. O. R. M. **THE PHARMACEUTICAL PERSPECTIVE IN ALZHEIMER'S DISEASE,** Porto, 2008.

LIMA J.S. **AGING, DEMENTIA AND ALZHEIMER'S DISEASE: WHAT DOES PSYCHOLOGY HAVE TO DO WITH IT?*,** Florianopolis - SC, Revista de Ciencias Humanas, n. 40, p. 469-489, 2006.

LOPES, A. J. ; PIROLO, N. D.; ARANDA, F. **ALZHEIMER'S DISEASE: NURSING CARING FOR THE CAREGIVER,** Londrina - PR, Revista saude, Vol. 15, Unpaginated, [2009].

PRADO, D.M.D. **GENETIC FACTORS INVOLVED IN ALZHEIMER'S DISEASE,** Porto, 2010.

RAMOS, D. A. ; RUAS, E. A. **ALZHEIMER'S DISEASE: LITERATURE REVIEW,** Apucarana - PR. Revista F@pciencia, v.11, n. 7, p. 44 - 53, 2017.

TRINDADE, E. B. N. **IMPORTANCE OF PHARMACEUTICAL ASSISTANCE FOR THE ELDERLY WITH ALZHEIMER'S DISEASE,** Goiarna - GO, Revista Especialize On-line IPOG, Vol. 01, Ano 8, Edi^ao n° 14 ,2017.

XIMENES, M.A. ; RICO, B.L.D. ; PEDREIRA, R.Q. **ALZHEIMER'S DISEASE: DEPENDENCY AND CARE,** Sao Paulo - SP, Revista Kairos Gerontologia, Vol. 17(2), p.121-140, 2014.

Chapter 9

MANAGEMENT AND PURCHASING IN HOSPITAL PHARMACY

Wellington de Paula[1] ; Josue Teixeira [1]; Michelle Melgarejo da Rosa[2]

1 - Pharmacy student at UniFBV Wyden University Centre

2 - Professor of Pharmacy at UniFBV Wyden University Centre

The presence of a hospital pharmacy department is of the utmost importance in every hospital. One of the aims of the department is to guarantee supply, reduce the excess of products and, consequently, reduce losses due to expiry. The purchase of medicines should take into account the necessary quantities of supplies, minimising purchases of medicines that are not needed and the appropriate quantity for use in a given period [1]. The choice of suppliers is an important issue for the smooth running of this sector within the hospital pharmacy, because if the supplier does not meet the specifications and pre-established dates, it can jeopardise the hospital's logistics, resulting in monetary losses, but above all, therapeutic losses (CRF-SP, 2010). In addition, the process of purchasing and acquiring medicines prevents medicines from being stored for longer than their expiry date, making it impossible to use them on patients (Pinto, 2016).

According to reports in the journal Farmacia Hospitalar[2] , in order to have better stock control in hospital pharmacies, certain points must be established, such as:

- Obtain products and services according to pre-scheduled consumption;

- Look for the same services and products at the lowest price;

- Check that the delivery is made in accordance with the type of material being delivered and that the packaging used preserves the quality of the product;

- Always maintain good communication with other sectors in order to see what can be saved and what can be improved in the supply of products and services;

The choice of supply involves the participation of various sectors in an organisation. After all, the medication must comply with criteria of effectiveness, quality, cost and safety, providing safe and rational conduct in the use of the medication that will be used in the institution.

[1] AЫOKЁA CASSIA PEREIRA SFORSIN; FABIO SENA DE SOUZA, MARISTELA BARROS DE SOUSA; NEUSSANA KELLEN DE ARAUJO MEDEIROS TORREAO; PAULO FREDERICO GALEMBECK; RENATA FERREIRA. Purchasing Management in Hospital   Pharmacy. Farmacia Hospitalar, Sao Paulo, Numero 16, pag. 3, March 2012.

[2] ANDRЁA CASSIA PEREIRA SFORSIN; FABIO SENA DE SOUZA, MARISTELA BARROS DE SOUSA; NEUSSANA KELLEN DE ARAUJO MEDEIROS TORREAO; PAULO FREDERICO GALEMBECK; RENATA FERREIRA. Purchasing Management in Hospital Pharmacy. Farmacia Hospitalar, Sao Paulo, Numero 16, pag. 3, March 2012.

Main parameters for product selection

The products that are part of the purchasing grid should be constantly evaluated, as it may happen that they are no longer produced, or are not being manufactured at the time of purchase (PAHO/WHO, 2015), or that they are no longer the prescriber's first choice, becoming a product out of use. As presentations and medicines are constantly being renewed, it is common for new products to appear and be added to the purchase list, with the aim of offering greater efficacy and fewer side effects, or providing the same efficacy as the product already in use, but at a lower cost.

Classification

The process of classifying medicines is in the form of coding for later consultation, making it easier to handle them in a way that minimises errors both for those who are going to use them and for those who are going to buy them (RDC №-157, OF 11 MAY 2017).

The way in which products are stored varies according to the establishment's methodology (clinics, hospitals, medical centres, etc.), as they can adopt either the criterion of storing products in alphabetical order or in pharmaceutical form. The most widely used in hospitals is the ABC curve of consumption or value (BARBIERI and MACHLINE, 2006), which consists of separating products according to their added value or consumption. Classification is important because if a particular medication is not available, it can be replaced by another of similar quality and efficacy.

Codified

This information is necessary to prevent errors from occurring, as it contains as much information as possible in order to reduce the possibility of errors. The coding process uses means of representation that vary in alphabetical, alphanumerical or numerical means (RDC №-157, OF 11 MAY 2017).

that a code never has more than one item and, likewise, that an item never has more than one code (Art. 6 of RDC 157/2017).

When and how much to buy

There are tools to help manage stock and demand. Of course, maintaining adequate stock control without technological resources would be time-consuming and involve a greater number of people. What's more, the losses and costs would be greater and would be attributable to hospital logistics. A demand survey, in this respect, must allow for the timely identification of the history of entries and exits, stock levels (minimum, maximum, resupply point), consumption data, met and unmet demand for each medicine, among other information that can be useful in the procurement process. Other relevant factors include medicines that are critical to purchase (exclusive suppliers and imported medicines) and seasonality, which causes fluctuations in the consumption of some medicines that can jeopardise the forecast.

You need a parameter of what is still in stock, what needs to be bought, avoiding high quantities due to poor stock planning (FERREIRA, 2002).

According to Wanke (2004), in order to have a stock with acceptable standards, certain requirements must be met.

1) Keeping the prices of each product up to date;

2) Establish parameters for the minimum and maximum quantities of stock that the hospital should have;

3) Keeping up to date with possible disuse of medication, avoiding its loss due to expiry;

4) Carry out frequent stock audits to check that the physical stock corresponds to the virtual stock;

5) Feed the stock management system with as much information as may be needed in the event of future queries, and check for possible errors in purchases;

6) Keeping strict control of everything that goes in and out of the hospital pharmacy's storage and dispensing sector.

Demand

Stock control is not an easy task, as it requires someone with experience and tools that can provide safe and efficient purchasing, because the best tools are no use if the operator doesn't have the minimum requirements to interpret the data. One of these is demand, which involves requirements that are often not found in the system's database, requiring a more comprehensive look. The Materials Requirements Planning spreadsheet system allows companies to calculate how much of a certain type of material is needed and at what time (PINHEIRO, 2001). It is a very complex system that requires countless controls and calculations of volume and time. Using the bibliographic reference as a basis, the ABC classification system was chosen to show the representativeness of each item in the stock as a whole, relating it to its demand. There are various types of demand, so it is important to know the existing demands and carry out an analysis to identify which of them the medicines available at the institution fall into (SANTOS et al., 2006).

- Permanent: These are products that have a long life and their purchase is based on the quantity necessary for the operation of the hospital, they are of constant use, that is, their concentrations must remain stable until the next purchase (e.g. serum, gloves, syringes, etc.);

- Specific, these are products in which demand increases according to the period of the year, also known as seasonality, because their movement varies according to the period of the year, being systematic, but not necessarily regular, also coming from natural causes, economic, rational and so on (e.g. medicines for asthma, measles, colds and so on).

- Irregular, they depend on other factors, such as promotion, marketing, etc. (e.g. most of the products come from prevention or control).

ABC curve

It is a method of classifying information. Products are analysed according to their class. Class A: the most important or value-added products, which are fewer in number but high in value, and are classified as the most valuable and profitable in the organisation's turnover (LOUREN£O et al., 2006). Class A products are linked to a large volume of resources. Even though they represent around 20% of an organisation's items, they account for a total of 80% of the total value of stock (OSMO, 2008). Ex: Antineoplastics.

Class B products are intermediate products, as they lie between classes A and C, representing around 15% of the total number of products in stock and consuming around 15% of resources (OSMO, 2008). E.g. antibiotics.

Class C represents around 70% of stock and is made up of items of lesser importance (not necessarily the cheapest), compromising only 20% of sample resources (OSMO, 2008). Items classified in class C can be worked on with a longer lead time, as their value has less impact on resources and they can be stocked in greater quantities (OSMO, 2008). E.g. serum. Syringes, bandages, adhesive plaster, etc.

On the other hand, we can also take into account other analyses, following certain principles, using the great importance of the items as a parameter, following the XYZ model, as shown below (TAKAHASHI 2008):

X- Represents products that can be substituted, and their lack does not represent a deviation in quality. For example, antibiotics.

Y- Represents products that can be replaced, but their lack represents a deviation in quality. Example: suture thread, the thickness of the thread influences quality.

Z- Cannot be replaced and its lack represents something that could delay a procedure, because even if it is something of low value, the procedure could not be completed if it were missing. An example is surgical gloves.

Suppliers:

It is a very important part of the hospital management process, and the right thing to do is not to get stuck with just a few suppliers, as this would imply possible supply disruptions, as well as limiting your mix to the products you work with. A good partnership for the supply of medicines is not just about the supplier having products and an attractive price, but also about after-sales service, as there will always be problems, which always happen (Ministerio da Saude, 2006). Reliability is extremely important, it guarantees commitment to the organisation and the quality of the products.

Management

Indicators are one of the most important tools in hospital management performance. They help to control and plan activities (CIPRIANO SL. 2009).

When, for some reason, this control breaks down, emergency orders are placed with partner pharmacies, which deliver the medication in a timely manner and with quality, in which case the amount to be paid is slightly higher than that bought from the usual suppliers (CIPRIANO, 2009).

REFERENCES

Pharmaceutical Assistance for Municipal Managers, Nelly Marin, PAHO/WHO, Rio de Janeiro, 2003.

SANTOS, G. A. A. Gestao de Farmacia Hospitalar. Sao Paulo: Ed. Senac, 2006.

PAN-AMERICAN HEALTH ORGANISATION. Brazilian consensus on pharmaceutical care: proposal. Brasilia, 2002. Available at: <http://bvsms.saude.gov.br/bvs/ publicacoes/PropostaConsensoAtenfar.pdf>. Accessed on: 25 August 2016.

Pan American Health Organisation/World Health Organisation (PAHO/WHO) in Brazil, 2015.

MLO NOVAES, AA GONCALVES, VMM SIMONETTI - XIII SIMPEP. Sao Paulo, 2006.

Sforsin ACP, Souza FS, Sousa MB et al. Purchasing management in hospital pharmacy. Farmacia Hospitalar [internet]. n° 16 mar^o/abril/maio 2012 [cited on 24 feb 2015).

Serrano RMSM, Masculo FS. Acquisition and storage of medicines by public health services [Internet]. 2001 Oct [cited 2015 Feb 18]. Available from: < http://www.abepro.org.br/biblioteca/enegep2001_tr10_0974.pdf > VALERY, P. P. T., Good practices for storing medicines. Brasilia: Central de Medicamentos, 1989. 22 p. http://www.abepro.org.br/biblioteca/enegep2001_tr10_0974.pdf. Accessed on: 16 May 2016.

Gomes MJVM, Reis AMM. Pharmaceutical sciences: An approach to hospital pharmacy. Sao Paulo; Atheneu, 2001.

WANKE, Peter . Trends in Inventory Management in Healthcare Organisations. Centre for

Logistics Studies - COPPEAD/UFRJ. Rio de Janeiro, 2004. Available at:http://www.centrodelogistica.com.br/new/fs-busca.htm?fr-art_saude.htm. Accessed on 25th March 2007.

PINHEIRO, Antonio Candido, LERNER, Eloi. TGCC: Implementation of an inventory control system in a commercial establishment - Case study - Santa Maria: UFSM, 2001.

SANTOS, AM; RODRIGUES, IA. Controlling Materials with Different Demand Patterns - A Case Study in a Chemical Industry. Management and Production. V.13, n. 2, p. 223231, 2006.

QUEIROZ, AA; CARVALHEIRO, D. Demand Forecasting and Seasonality Detection Method for Production Planning in Food Industries. XXIII .

OSMO, F.P.F.; OSMO, A.A. Supply management and hospital costs. "In" STORPIRTS, S; et al. Farmacia Clinica e Aten^ao Farmaceutica. Rio de Janeiro: Guanabara Koogan, 2008b.

TAKAHASHI, P.S.K.; RIBEIRO, E. Acquisition of medicines and materials. "In" STORPIRTS, S; et al. Farmacia Clinica e Aten^ao Farmaceutica. Rio de Janeiro: Guanabara Koogan, 2008b.

Brazil. Ministry of Health. Secretariat for Science, Technology and Strategic Inputs. Department of Pharmaceutical Assistance and Strategic Inputs. Acquisition of medicines for pharmaceutical assistance in the SUS: basic guidelines - Brasilia: Ministry of Health, 2006. 56 p.

CIPRIANO SL. Development of a model for the construction and application of a set of performance indicators in hospital pharmacy with a focus on comparability. Sao Paulo; 2009. Doctoral dissertation - Faculty of Public Health, University of Sao Paulo

Chapter 10

THE INDISCRIMINATE USE OF ANTIMICROBIALS IN HOSPITAL SETTINGS

Alberto Jose Santiago[1] ; Michelle Melgarejo da Rosa[2]

1 - Pharmacy student at UniFBV Wyden University Centre

2 - Professor of Pharmacy at UniFBV Wyden University Centre

For a long time, human beings have lived with the existence of various microorganisms on the earth's surface, and we suffer from the different pathologies they cause. This has led to the indiscriminate use of antimicrobials growing uncontrollably in hospital settings. In some cases, prescriptions are not based on clinical studies of patients, thus failing to follow all the rigour required by the Ministry of Health.

Another deficiency in clinical procedures is the lack of a hospital routine based on collective action by the multidisciplinary team, which could contribute to establishing guidelines that lead to the correct use of antimicrobials.

It is stated that: "the use of antimicrobials in hospitals contributes to the development of bacterial resistance, increasing hospital costs and the risks of adverse drug reactions" (BETOLOLI, 2010). This justifies the excessive use of these drugs as a public health problem.

Therefore, the purpose of this work is to describe what "antimicrobial drugs" are, their action on the human body, adverse reactions, their use in hospital methodologies, as well as theories that address and justify this topic.

MOST COMMONLY USED ANTIMICROBIALS IN HOSPITAL SETTINGS

Since ancient times, human health has been one of the most discussed topics by various researchers in the world of science, but over the years, as a result of the demand for diseases that have emerged in today's society, other forms of procedures to combat them have had to be implemented. As a result, other drugs have gained prominence in hospital environments, including antimicrobials.

According to ANVISA (2007), these medicines can be defined as: "a class of drugs that is frequently consumed in hospitals and in the community." In other words, they can be ingested both in public-private healthcare settings and in the community at large in pharmacies, with greater caution being exercised when they are administered in a hospital setting, due to the possible alteration of the microbial ecology that these medicines can cause.

In hospital settings, different antimicrobial drugs are prescribed on a daily basis, but according to a survey carried out by Geum magazine (Geum Newsletter) in 2015, the most prescribed class of drug was penicillins (40 per cent - Amoxicillin), administered in two ways: as a 7-day treatment (31.61) and as an oral suspension (100 per cent).

In another survey, carried out at the state hospital of Bahia, in the municipality of Jequie, in August 2015, in partnership with the Hospital Infection Control Commission (CCIH), it was found that among the most prescribed restricted-use antimicrobials, the combination of piperacillin/tazobacton (32%) and cefepine (28%) were the most prevalent.

According to this scenario, a survey carried out in a private hospital in the interior of Rio Grande do Sul highlighted that cephalosporins (43.4%), penicillins (16.3%) fluoroquinolones (13%) and aminoglycosides (9.7%) accounted for the majority of hospital use. This shows that antimicrobials are among the most widely used groups of drugs in Brazilian hospitals.

MICROBIAL RESISTANCE

It can be defined as the ability of microorganisms to develop more easily in the body. Microbial resistance is growing rapidly in hospital settings. Despite great advances in pharmaceuticals and medicine, these have not been enough to significantly minimise the use of antimicrobials in hospitals.

The mechanisms of microbial resistance are summarised as: a change in the permeability of the bacterial membrane, so the antibiotic cannot bind and exert its pharmacological effect; efflux of the antibiotic out of the bacteria, a mechanism carried out by bacterial enzymes; a change in the permeability of the antibiotic's binding site, which also prevents its effect; and most importantly for most antibiotics, resistance induced by bacterial enzymatic degradation.

It is important for health organisations to develop more effective methodologies to combat bacterial resistance. Some of these can be highlighted, such as: reducing the abusive use of antimicrobial drugs in hospital settings, not changing dosages, greater supervision and rigour in the administration of these drugs, developing new drugs and more competent vaccines, implementing measures to control hospital infections, among others. The indiscriminate use of antimicrobials in hospital and home environments increases the number of reported cases of bacterial resistance every year. Naturally, coupled with this high number, there are fewer pharmacological alternatives to infections and fewer chances of curing patients. Measures to promote the rational use of medicines, propaganda explaining bacterial resistance, hospital programmes and/or courses are some of the measures that can be implemented in this area.

ADVERSE REACTIONS

The most common adverse reactions to the use of antimicrobials are nausea, vomiting, abdominal pain, kidney problems, dizziness, lack of appetite, constipation, anorexia, among others. They can be conceptualised by the WHO as an adverse event or any unfavourable medical occurrence, which can happen during the administration of a certain drug, where this occurrence cannot necessarily be related to the process developed by the patient.

Most of these conditions can lead to patient morbidity and mortality. As a result, there is an increase in hospitalisation time, and consequently a rise in the cost of maintaining such treatments in public or private health institutes.

BISSON in 2007 reported that the majority of antimicrobial procedures are carried out excessively and inappropriately, leading to greater damage to the clinical state of the individuals being treated. In addition, other issues need to be addressed, such as poor administration of medication, length of hospitalisation, time away from school and work, disability or death, in other words, social and personal issues.

It is clear that physical, psychological, emotional and social issues make certain patients possibly more vulnerable to micro-organisms, because during most of these periods, their immunity is low, making it necessary for the whole hospital team to intervene immediately to find possible solutions to these problems.

The importance of more rigorous and effective methodologies in clinical procedures is an immediate necessity. Different drugs were highlighted, as they are the most commonly used in hospitals, as well as problems such as resistance and adverse effects that can be caused by them. It is quite convincing to emphasise the statement by FERRAZ, 2014:

"The joint action of the pharmacist with the entire medical team, to carry out active searches and internal audits of antimicrobial prescribing, leads to improvements in the standards of antibiotic prescribing."

In this way, there will be a lower rate of drug poisoning and greater efficiency in eradicating the various infections that occur in hospital environments, thus preserving both the clinical condition of patients and their professional ethical identity.

Therefore, the use of antimicrobials is essential in hospital treatment, but clinical diagnostics must be carried out to show the entire therapeutic status of patients, as well as being prescribed in accordance with the rigour determined by the Brazilian Ministry of Health, so that public health can significantly benefit the lives of citizens.

REFERENCES

ANDRADE, Denize. **Occurrence of Multiresistant Bacteria in an Intensive Care Centre of a Brazilian Emergency Hospital**. Brazilian Intensive Care Journal: Sao Paulo, 2006.

ARIEL, Ricardo. **Indiscriminate Use of Antimicrobials and Microbial Resistance N°03**. Horus: Brasilia, 2016.

ATHAYDE, Fernanda. **Profile of Antimicrobial Use in a Private Hospital**. Scielo Saude Publica: Porto Alegre, 2006.

FANHANI, Helen. **Inadequate Use of Cephalosporins and the Role of the Hospital Infection Control Committee**. Revista Saude e Biologia: Campo Grande, 2011.

FERREIRA, Ilara. **Problems Related to Antimicrobials in an Intensive Care Unit at a Public Hospital in Teresina**. UFP: Teresina, 2011.

GOMES, Ramon. **Prescribing Antimicrobials for Restricted Use in Patients Admitted to a Teaching Hospital**. Brazilian Journal of Hospital Pharmacy: Sao Paulo, 2016.

KAPOSAKI, Liria. **Analysis of the Use and Bacterial Resistance to Antimicrobials at Hospital Level**. Brazilian Journal of Pharmacy: Sao Paulo, 2012.

LOURO, Ricardo. **Adverse Events to Antibiotics in Patients Admitted to a University Hospital**. Revista Saude Publica: Maringa, 2007.

LUCAS, Jose. **Profile of Paediatric Antimicrobial Prescriptions Dispensed in a Basic Pharmacy in the Interior of Ceara**. Geum: Rainha do Sertao, 2015.

LUZ, Silvania. **Evaluation of the Use of Antibiotics in a Philanthropic Hospital in the Municipality of Bage - RS**. UFP: Rio Grande do Sul, 2014.

MONTE, Lidiane. **Indiscriminate Use of Antibiotics and Microbial Resistance: A Reflection on the Treatment of Hospital Infections**. NOVAFAPI Interdisciplinary Journal: Teresina, 2011.

MOREIRA, Leila. **Principles for the Rational Use of Antimicrobials**. AMRIGS Magazine: Porto Alegre, 2004.

RIBEIRO, Romario. **Rational Use of Antimicrobials**. PUC: Goias, 2015.

ROCHA, Marco. **Study of the Use of Antimicrobial Medicines from 2003 to 2004 in Adult Patients in a Tertiary Hospital in Rio de Janeiro**. Revista Brasileira de Farmacia: Rio de Janeiro,

2009.

SANTOS, Rafael. **Consequences of Excessive Use of Antimicrobials in Postoperative Care: The Context of a Public Hospital**. Revista Col. Brasileira: Brasilia, 2014.

VAZ, Douglas. **The Use of Antimicrobials in the Hospital Environment and the Pharmacist's Duties in the Hospital Infection Control Committee (CCIH)**. Fasem: Goias, 2014.

WANNMACHER, Lenita. **Indiscriminate Use of Antibiotics and Microbial Resistance: A Lost War? Rational Use of** Medicines. Selected Topics: Maringa, 2004.

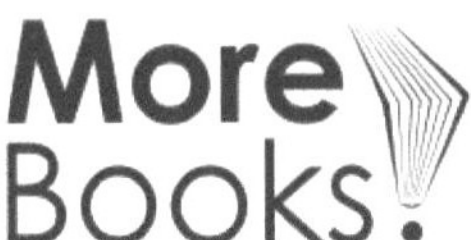

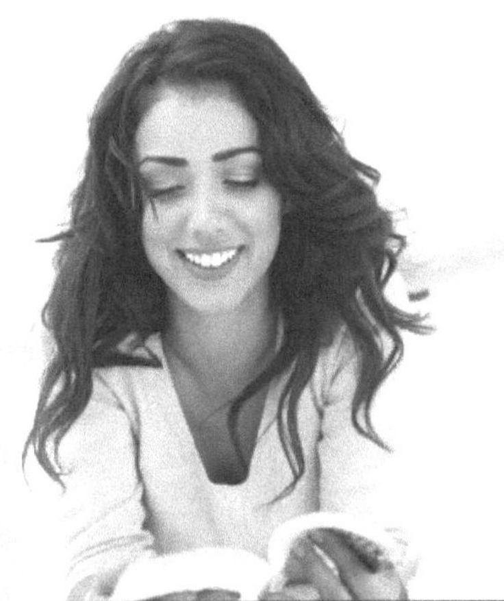

I want morebooks!

Buy your books fast and straightforward online - at one of world's fastest growing online book stores! Environmentally sound due to Print-on-Demand technologies.

Buy your books online at
www.morebooks.shop

Kaufen Sie Ihre Bücher schnell und unkompliziert online – auf einer der am schnellsten wachsenden Buchhandelsplattformen weltweit! Dank Print-On-Demand umwelt- und ressourcenschonend produzi ert.

Bücher schneller online kaufen
www.morebooks.shop

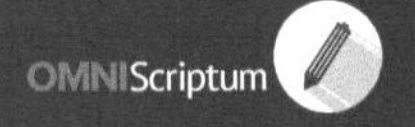

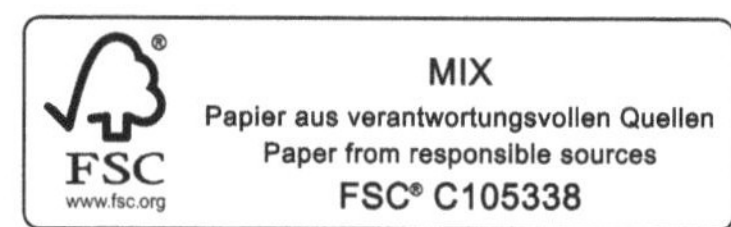

Printed by Books on Demand GmbH, Norderstedt / Germany